# Ethereal Crystal Healing

"Marie Delanote's book about ethereal crystals will teach and assist you. The timing for this book is perfect. Her wisdom and experience as an ethereal crystals master is beyond anyone else. She is the best teacher leading the way in this new energy field."

~ **Dame Marie Diamond,** master teacher in the global phenomena *The Secret,* mariediamond.com

"I love Marie's work. Her work with the ethereal crystals has supported me in so many ways, and her personal advice has been so valuable. Working with the ethereal crystals has brought real positive transformation in my energy."

~ **Annette Dernick,** speaker and coach for Love and Peace in Companies, author of *Der Peace Faktor*

"Ethereal crystals are great to use with babies and children, and very much so with those with special needs. I find they respond very well and make great progress, often unexpectedly, such as being able to tune into others and communicate more effectively. Very suitable for animals as well—including those who mistrust people."

~ **Niamh Horgank,** special needs teacher

# Ethereal Crystal Healing

## Create Your Life with the Frequencies of Stones

### Marie Delanote

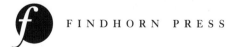

FINDHORN PRESS

Findhorn Press
One Park Street
Rochester, Vermont 05767
www.findhornpress.com

Findhorn Press is a division of Inner Traditions International

**Disclaimer**
The information in this book is given in good faith and intended for information
only. Neither author nor publisher can be held liable by any person for any loss
or damage whatsoever which may arise from the use of this book or any of the
information therein.

Cataloging-in-Publication data for this title is available from the Library of Congress

ISBN 979-8-88850-016-3 (print)
ISBN 979-8-88850-017-0 (ebook)

Printed and bound in China by Reliance Printing Co., Ltd.

10 9 8 7 6 5 4 3 2 1

Edited by Nicky Leach
Text design and layout by Anna-Kristina Larsson
This book was typeset in Garamond, Spartan and Itangiuh

To send correspondence to the author of this book, mail a first-class letter
to the author c/o Inner Traditions • Bear & Company, One Park Street,
Rochester, VT 05767, USA and we will forward the communication,
or contact the author directly at **www.mariedelanote.net**.

# Contents

**PART TWO**

# 33 Ethereal Crystals and Their Healing Powers

**PART THREE**
# Healing with Ethereal Crystals

# Preface

We all have family lines. Whether you were adopted and have no idea where you come from, or whether you are fully aware of all the shenanigans in your family, you don't need to know what happened in your past to transform your life. You just need to be accountable, look yourself truly in the mirror, and get going!

I did some digging in my own family line, and what I found was very interesting.

My paternal grandfather lost his father as a child right after his youngest brother was born. They were wealthy West Flemish (Belgian) farmers, but after my great-grandfather died, my great-grandmother had to look after seven children and a big farm all by herself.

Remarkably, my grandmother also lost her father as a child. Just like my other great-grandparents, they were wealthy people, who owned a big bleach company in West Flanders. When my great-grandfather died, the company went bankrupt and my great-grandmother had to do everything she could to survive and support her three daughters.

A strong vibration of women "doing it all"—tough, heroic, and survivors—emanates from my father's line. Both of my father's parents experienced a huge shift in financial circumstances while growing up as a result of their father's death, so wealth and status were of central concern to them their whole lives.

My grandfather became a highly successful bank director and director of retirement homes, and as a result, my grandmother was able to restore her status generously thanks to him. The fear of losing everything left a huge imprint on my grandparents, though, and I remember vividly how my grandmother would hide cash under her mattress and in her corset before going to visit "the cathedrals".

"The cathedrals" was just another way of saying "the banks of Luxembourg", where they brought their money to avoid paying taxes. But now I know that that money must have been black market money, and God knows how it was earned—a deal here and there under the table, easy money for a rainy day. My paternal grandparents were an affluent couple with huge fears of losing their money or being betrayed. My grandmother didn't trust anyone.

On my mother's side, my great-grandmother was from the French-speaking part of Belgium, back when it was the wealthy part of the country, while my great-grandfather was from the Flemish part, the poor part of Belgium. Their first son, my grandfather, was born less than nine months after they got married. It is believed that they got married because she was pregnant and, because of the times, she had to move to Flanders to be with her new husband and family.

My grandfather and great-grandmother had a love–hate relationship throughout his life; she seems to have blamed her son for having to get married and move to the "poor" part of the country. He went on to become a successful doctor, but worked long hours his whole life to prove his worth to his loved ones, apparently in response to this love–hate relationship with his mother, whom he could never please.

My maternal great-grandfather had a small confectionery business. His own brother stole money from him, and the business eventually went bankrupt. My grandmother was a quiet woman, who suffered her husband's pain in silence. To this day, I can hear him reciting his motto "Work, work, work!" even as she organized everything behind the scenes.

Both my grandparents on my mother's side lived through World War II. As young adults, they were actively involved in the resistance in Belgium, and he was captured once. As an 18-year-old, my grandmother hid messages in her underwear and cycled through German posts—you can only imagine what would have happened to her if she had been caught. This is only the tip of the iceberg of what they did for their country during the war, and the fear they carried with them.

My mother and father have a whole story of their own. My father left when I was five, remarried, this time to a wealthy woman, and also had an illegitimate child who died at just nine months old. Meanwhile, my mother worked all hours to support her four daughters and keep her own head above water emotionally.

And then there is me. I am the result of all that has happened in my family line before me (as are you)—in my case, a woman thinking that she has to "do it all" alone, who is tough, a survivor. As with so many of us, I'm an old soul, carrying vibrations within me that are hundreds, even thousands, of years old.

As a young child, I felt stupid, unworthy, and unsupported by life and family; in my dreams, in my heart, I wanted to stand on stage, be seen, be out there, be successful, and make a real difference. So I wrote a book called "The Magic Pill" and that magic pill was for me—a pill that made me smart in a second, that made sure I was seen, heard, and successful with one snap of the finger.

I was carrying the vibration of the women in my family who always ended up having to do everything themselves because men left (whether that was through death or not). I carried the vibration of my mother's parents of not trusting people and a constant feeling of not being safe, which they experienced during the second world war. I carried the vibration of having to work extremely hard to be noticed. Finally, I carried the vibration that money runs out, because of my paternal grandparents' family businesses going under after their fathers died and my other grandmother's father's business going bankrupt after his own family cheated on him.

My little book solved all those issues in a second. It made me smart, loved, rich, seen, heard, and successful. Back then, I had no idea about my family's background. All I knew was how I was feeling and experiencing life, and I wanted it to be different.

Who can relate to that?

My "magic pill" wasn't some childish hallucination. It really is possible. We don't even need a pill for it. That magic pill simply is a new vibration.

This book, *Ethereal Crystals,* is the essence of everything I learned and now teach the world. It is my mission to help you and humanity to ascend the human consciousness and vibration, because when we do that, magical things unfold, and we can create every little detail of the life we dream of.

I'll try to help you answer the following questions:

- How do I change the physical world I experience?
- How do I lift my vibration and that of others?
- How do I create perfect health, happiness, love, success, and abundance?

My book will help you look at things differently, more openly. It will help you realize that you are the core of your own existence, the source of all creation—both for yourself and for the collective through your vibration.

My book will help you see the magic within you—the oneness, the wholeness. I often hear from people, "Wow, those ethereal crystals! This is completely new. I have never heard of this before." Once they find out more, they are blown away and start creating their own life, allowing health, happiness, love, and abundance into their life. I hope this happens for you too. Everything starts right here, right now, with you.

Welcome to the world of ethereal crystals.

# Part One

# The Dimension of the Ethereal Crystals

# Mother Earth's Crystals

## Acknowledging Mother Earth's Precious Gems

Ethereal crystals are vibrational tools created for humanity to help raise its frequency and assist in the ascension of human consciousness. This book aims to bring in an awareness of these vibrational crystals and thus foster enlightenment while also helping you to raise your vibration and to create a life of health, happiness, success, and abundance.

Before I talk further about ethereal crystals though, I must acknowledge Mother Earth's gorgeous physical crystals! They have looked after us and taught us so much for millions of years. Learning about ethereal crystals will never diminish the value of physical crystals, only help them and us for the better.

We all know about the gorgeous colourful minerals formed underground in Mother Earth's belly, the gems or crystals. For some people, crystals are just beautiful stones, but for many, crystals help make things better—physically, emotionally, and mentally.

Everything in this physical world vibrates: very low, low, mid, high, very high. That is a scientific fact. It is the same with crystals. They vibrate at a certain frequency and affect everything and everyone around them.

Crystals vibrate energy within Mother Earth and out into the world, nature, and the consciousness of the people living where the crystals are, and beyond. Thanks to the beautiful gift that crystals give us, humans can raise their vibration, and this affects everything they do for themselves and others. It is a forever expanding game.

Crystals are mined globally and sold as rough or polished crystals, or they are made into jewellery, lamps, and even furniture so that people can enjoy their healing powers in whatever way they wish. What is not thought through, though, is that the moment crystals are taken out of Mother Earth their vibration changes.

They are affected by:

- The vibration of the human removing the crystal
- The machinery
- The sun's UV rays
- Being transported! Most crystals travel so many miles, it adds to global warming when their main job is to help the planet, not destroy it.

By the time our precious crystals get to us, their vibration has diminished dramatically. By being removed from the place where they belong, the vibrational balance has changed, negatively affecting the planet, nature, animals, and humans.

I love physical crystals. They are so beautiful and invaluable. They have also brought us so much knowledge in the times that humans needed physical and tactile solutions for their healing. But times are changing, and people are starting to realize that we must do things differently in order to save the planet and humanity. We can't bury our heads in the sand. We must open our eyes.

Physical crystals represent:

- The old consciousness.
- Attachment to the world of physical limitations.
- Value to the planet and humans as long as they stay in Mother Earth.

Ethereal crystals represent:

- The new consciousness.
- Going beyond anything we've ever experienced, breaking our glass ceiling.
- Value to the expansion of human consciousness and vibration.

We are ready to move from the physical world to the vibrational world now that our consciousness has grown and our awareness expanded. Vibration is our source, the roots of all we experience during this physical existence.

So let me introduce you to the vibrant world of ethereal crystals! Ethereal crystals are nonmaterial; that is, they do not exist physically as crystals but as pure vibration that you can tap into simply by using your intention. Ethereal crystals are a reminder of the power within, how all healing, happiness, and abundance already lives within you.

Ethereal crystals are some four hundred times stronger than those found on Earth, because they are pure, come directly from the Universe, and have never been handled by humans. Anyone can tap into the infinite high vibration of ethereal crystals because we are all connected to everything and everyone, in all directions of time and space. They are here to support us in our further expansion and ascension of our human mind and vibration.

The world is changing, and as we live in the Aquarius era, we're focusing more on the fact that everything is vibration and everything is connected. We're going back to the source of everything: vibration and oneness. Now is the time to work with the pure vibration of ethereal crystals.

Imagine walking through life and with one thought: healing, changing, creating, and transforming—allowing Mother Earth, nature, animals, and humans to thrive and raise their consciousness and vibrations.

# Understanding Vibration
## Vibration Is at the Core
## of Our Existence

You have already heard me talk about vibration several times. That is because vibration is the core of our existence. Without it, the world as we know it wouldn't be possible.

I could talk about the Big Bang, but I won't. I have no knowledge in the matter, and it is just another way of trying to understand the beginning of ourselves.

People have this innate need to understand "the beginning". They are so attached to the physical world, they need to understand every beginning and every end. Everything must have a touchable explanation. In thinking this way, we stay stuck within the boundaries of our known world and hold ourselves back from riding the wave of expansion. This shows that we do not trust our true nature, which is limitless.

What if there is no beginning and no end, only expansion? If there is expansion, it follows that there must have been a beginning. An expansive universe is just another way to try and understand things. Everything any human could ever think of is already here, just waiting to be noticed.

How does it get noticed?

It gets noticed by the expansion of human consciousness. This is a very different thing, as it is not the universe that expands but human consciousness, allowing us to notice all that is, thus creating fabulous physical experiences and making its journey back to the source of all that is—the unlimited universe.

Scientists have been able to record sounds in the universe. We can hear those sounds as they are created by vibration. Everything in life starts with vibration. It is the vibration that creates a certain energy. It is the energy that determines the physical outcome. Depending on the tones we hear, they were created by different vibrations.

Think about when you meet someone new and say, "Oh, yes, we're vibing." What does that mean? It means you're on the same wavelength, you understand each other, you feel each other. Or it might be the opposite. "Gosh, we really weren't vibing." That's because you're on a different wavelength.

Think about it. When you were vibing (or not), and someone asks what caused it, you might say, "I don't know. It just didn't feel right. It felt weird." We're going into that feeling.

The vibe we're feeling is a nonphysical experience. At the source of everything lies exactly that, the vibe. It is a nonphysical explanation of whether it fits you or not. You walk into a room, and you feel that it's not comfortable. That is the energy you can feel, created by a vibration—a mindset, emotions, words, happenings. Just like animals, we pick up on them with our nonphysical receptors.

Low vibrations come from swear words, ugly words, emotional pain, physical attack, doubt, shame, guilt. High vibrations come from laughter, love (the highest vibration of all), beautiful words, excitement, happiness, trust. As you speak, feel, and act, you create. As you feel other vibrations and react to them, you create.

For example, say someone is organizing a party for you and shows everything on a mood board. You favour black, heavy metal, and outdoor parties, but the organizer presents you with a mood board showing plans for an indoor, pink, fluffy unicorn party. You will most likely mention that you were after another vibe! In this case, the party organizer got the vibe wrong. Colours and sounds all have a different vibration, which creates a particular kind of energy and specific physical results. We react to vibrations emotionally and physically.

Imagine sand on a plate. As we turn on music, the sand will form a pattern depending on the vibration of the music. It starts with a vibration and creates a physical form. But do you know that we don't have to hear or see vibration for it to be real? Everything vibrates, whether we can see it or not. Even the sand grains and rocks on the beach vibrate.

Imagine now that one of your friends is in a bad mood. You're around them all day, as you live together, so there is a strong chance that her mood will affect you. Do you know the expression "If you lie down with dogs, you will get up with fleas"? It refers to being aware of who and what you surround yourself with. It's all vibration affecting you and everything around it. This is why lifting your vibration is important, as it helps you create new physical environments and experiences. On top of that, as we are all connected, your vibration will positively affect you and everything and everyone around you.

Without vibration, there is no energy. Without energy, there is no physical world, no physical existence. Everything you see in your physical world exists because it vibrates. Without the vibration, it wouldn't exist. The physical world is there as an expression of vibration.

Raising vibration is exactly what we're doing when working with ethereal crystals as their vibrations are super high! Why is it good to raise your vibration?

1　You will rise above physical and psychological illnesses and diseases.
2　You will create more happiness in your life.
3　You will attract more success, serendipity, luck, "coincidences", love, and abundance in your life.
4　You will create the life you truly desire.
5　You will inspire others to do the same, as you will be giving off this vibration, affecting everything and everyone around you.
6　By raising your vibration, you will be helping the ascension of human consciousness and vibration, saving the planet and humanity.

Let's raise our vibrations!

# No Time, No Space

## Acknowledging Our Unlimited Being

As humans, we struggle to think of ourselves without limits because we experience ourselves as being in a two-dimensional not a three-dimensional world. Everything we see with our physical eyes has a beginning and an end—nothing is limitless; everything has a positive and a negative pole. Growing up, we are programmed to hear and see how something starts and ends, is good or bad, sweet or sour, hot or cold, positive or negative.

We need to reprogramme our mind to understand that we are limitless. Our natural state is perfect health, perfect happiness, perfect abundance. This is hard to know with your brain, so you must believe it with your mind. There is no such thing as time and space, so unless you change things, the vibrations you are sending out right now will continue into the future, creating the same old physical experiences.

Time is linear: everything happens right now. You are who you are because of all the vibrations you carry with you in your conscious thinking, subconscious thinking, your aura (energy field around you), your mind, and your chakras (energy portals in and around your body). Everything that ever happened to you has added to a certain vibration you are sending out right now. That vibration is what determines what you see around you, your physical state, and how you experience your life.

Time is the biggest illusion every human on this planet has collectively created. The universe is boundless. There is no separation, no boundaries, no time or opposites.

You are an accumulation of everything and everyone that has ever happened to you until you become aware and change that vibration. As that happens, you change your energy, and with that, you change your physical experiences.

It happens instantly and ripples out like a pebble that has been thrown in a pond. The only thing that stops the physical change is the stubbornness of humans that has them return again and again to their old vibrational habits. This can keep people stuck for tens, hundreds, or thousands of years. You need to be persistent.

Humans actually get the chance to work through their limiting beliefs, strained connections, pain, and stubborn habits after they pass away. When you die, you enter what we call "a waiting room", where you are surrounded by your guides and the highest of Universal beings. In that moment, you revisit your whole life and even feel how others have felt as a result of your actions. In the waiting room, you have the opportunity to learn, heal, and progress before you come back and continue to evolve. You get the chance to heal karma, your fate in future existences as an effect of past actions. Unfortunately, many souls are so excited to come back, that they do not fully complete that level. This results in many returning souls falling straight back into their old habits, connections . . . vibration. Luckily, the ethereal crystals can help us heal karma whilst living life.

If you want a new story, you need a new vibration. Everything you no longer want is your old story. You are still sitting in your chair reading a book you created when you were a slave. Put the book down. There is only now. What is your new story? Let's start with a matching vibration, and the new story will follow.

Everything your soul has ever experienced was signposted from your conscious to your subconscious mind and programmed in your subconscious mind. There is only now, so unless your sometimes inexplicable fears, habits, pain are consciously addressed, they will continue to be sent out as vibrations into your world, and more of the same vibrations will be boomeranged straight back to you. It is a never-ending circle. You, and only you, can change that. Vibrations never go away, but they can be instantly changed in any number of ways. Your story is attached to your vibration; your vibration is attached to your story.

I say your vibration is "boomeranged back" because like attracts like. Imagine two horizontal lines. The bottom line will never meet the top line, and the top line will never meet the bottom line; unless, that is, we move the bottom line on top of the top line, then they become one. And that can only happen when we lift the bottom line.

Like attracts like. High vibrations are matched with high vibrations. Low vibrations are matched with low vibrations. If you're on the lower line, you'll have to move to the higher line to receive what's there.

Physical and emotional experiences that match lower vibrations:

- Depression
- Disease
- Illness
- Doubts
- Guilt
- Fear
- Money issues
- Emotional pain
- Bad relationships
- Unpleasant house and neighbourhood
- Painful/unpleasant environment

Physical experiences that match higher vibrations:

- Flow of life
- Ease of life
- Fabulous relationships
- Money flow and abundance
- Honesty
- Trust
- Happiness
- Success

Imagine: You roll in the mud and are covered in dirt, but you also want to go to that chic party. But even though you want it so badly—you belong there, you have the talent to be there, and your soul must be there—there is no way they will let you come in looking so dirty. Unless, that is, you wash the dirt off. When you wash it off, you attract what you want: You look clean, smell nice, and present like everyone else, or better, so they allow you in. Unless you wash that dirt off, you will stay dirty and will not be invited in.

It's the same with the vibrations you carry. Unless you change vibrations, they stick around. Unless you change those vibrations that are stopping you from reaching your new story, you will remain out of vibration with what you want. Remember, like attracts like. Everything will continue until you change the vibration. When you change the vibration, you'll get different results.

Imagine: In a past life, you were burnt at the stake as a witch. The fear of performing alternative healing now vibrates in your aura, your chakras, and your subconscious mind, and leads you to avoid performing healing work openly and keep safely hidden from others to protect yourself from being "killed" for it. If that energy actively vibrates, no matter how much you now, in this life, want the outside world to notice you, they won't, because you vibrate "fear of being seen"; that is, unless you change that vibration.

A long time ago, when I was living in a new town and visited local shops to drop-off flyers so people would know about the healing sessions I provided, I was terrified. I felt so scared, my hands were sweaty, I was flustered, and my voice trembled. My body went into fight-or-flight mode. Even though I badly wanted to get new clients, the vibration I was giving off said something completely different and not one client came from distributing those flyers. The energy I was giving off was my old story; to create my new story, I had to change my vibration. Which I did!

Imagine: You lost loved ones in past lives or this life and grieved deeply and never got over it. That pain and fear to feel it again is carried in your subconscious mind, your aura, and chakras; it is in your vibration. This is a type of blockage that blocks the sacral and heart chakras which, if not healed and dealt with, can cause further blockage and lead to physical illness, such as issues with the lungs; breast, ovarian, or uterine cancer; heart disease; and so on. Unless, that is, the vibration is changed. The physical body cannot create this by itself; it reacts to the vibration.

Imagine: You are a woman and your father is a Don Juan—he has married three times and still sleeps around. As a girl, you wouldn't consciously have known this, but vibrationally you picked that up and programmed it as your own. Once you become an adult, unless healing takes place, you are likely to carry the belief that men cheat. Since you are giving off that vibration, there is a strong chance that your partner will be sexually promiscuous and have a wandering eye or cheat on you, or you will have lifelong trust issues. Unless, that is, you become aware and change the vibration!

When you think about what you want but your vibration says something else, you are stopping yourself from receiving what you desire. It is like trying to drive an old rusty car that has been left untouched in the shed for 40 years. No matter how hard you try, the car will have difficulty starting or won't start at all. After some much-needed love and attention—changing the oil, cleaning the pipes, replacing a few bits—the car will drive. It's the equivalent of changing vibration for humans.

Change those old vibrations to liberate yourself. Once those old vibrational patterns, beliefs, and events have been changed, the energy changes and as a result, it is a whole lot easier to apply positive thinking and abundant living. When those old vibrations—sometimes a thousand years old or more—are gone, the Universe can no longer match them as they are not there, so everything happens in the here and now. At that point, it will be easy to move forward and concentrate on the beautiful life of love, health, and abundance you wish for.

To acknowledge your unlimited nature, you really do only need to look at your own life. Your life has nothing to do with anyone else but your own vibration. You might want to blame your father, your grandmother, or your friend for the misfortunes you experience. The truth is, this happened because it's in your vibration. Let it go, forgive others, send love, and forgive yourself for having allowed that lower vibration in.

There was a moment in time when all you were was a vibrational thought. Whether that came from one or two parents, or from your own soul present in another dimension or time or space, that vibration created energy, and all the specifics of soul contracts, past vibrations, lessons, spider webs of connections, created the perfect combination of an egg and a sperm. As these two melted together, that initial thought of life became physical. That was your first evolution of limitlessness.

You continued to expand into a human being, with intellect, physical capabilities, and other qualities, the direct result of the vibration that was present. You expanded into a breathing and living human baby, then further expanded into a critically thinking, loving toddler, teenager, and adult. You can continue learning and expanding forever. It will take you as far as your consciousness allows, depending on whether you accept new vibrations, consciousness, and so on coming into this life.

On the soul level, you accept expansion every time; on the human level, it might take you five, ten, a thousand, ten thousand lives to accept it. But that's a different story. The fact that you're reading this book shows huge expansion and collaboration in the growth of humanity to a whole new level. As a consciousness, we simply need to remember our limitlessness and oneness and be accountable for our own expansion.

It might blow your mind when I mention that there is no time or space. After all, we see touchable, physical things all around us. We go from A to B and deal with time, delay, movement, and it all appears so real, right?

The best explanation I can give is to imagine that you are inside a computer and that you are in that big black screen. As you're in that computer, in that infinite black space, you also see little blue specks. When you touch them, you receive information. You touch more specks; you receive more information depending on what specks you touch. All the information you asked your computer 10 years ago is there. All the information you ask your computer today is there. All the information you will ask your computer in 20 years will be there so is already there now. This is part of the evolution of the computer. It is all in there; it is ready. All you need to do is be aware of it, click the specks, and *boom*, there is the information you wanted.

Your great-grandparents might not know how to do it, because they were born in a different era, so they don't understand it, and this is the equivalent of a different consciousness. But still, it already exists, whether they understand it or not.

Everything exists now. Everything we experience now that wasn't physically present 20 years ago was still already there. Everything that will be physically detectable in 150 years cannot be seen yet but is already present. This is evolution of the understanding of the unlimited black screen. We ask, it is answered, and as the knowledge of limitlessness and the here and now within the human consciousness expands, we receive more answers to our questions. It is already here; it just needs a human consciousness, awareness, intention, to click on it and bring it into physical reality.

There is no time. There is no space. There is only now. Everything is here, all the time. There is only the human consciousness that decides it's ready, and to use it in this physical world.

This is also how psychics work. This is how people look beyond the veil. They just click the specks in the black computer screen and ask for information. We can walk into a room and feel what happened there when we click the specks. When we ask a question, we receive the vibration. The vibration is the answer, which we then translate into images, words, feelings, and reality. I am my ancestors; we are one. I expand; they expand. This can all be done with raising vibration, using the vibration of ethereal crystals. We're adding that knowledge, that information, into the human consciousness. We expand for ourselves and for everyone else now.

# 4

# Aquarius Time

## Grasping the Need to Work with Ethereal Crystals

### *The Aquarius Era*
*The time when humans take control of their destiny
by expanding their consciousness*

Humanity is at a crucial point. There is a lot of talk about whether the planet and the human species will survive or not. Many previous civilizations also came to this same crossroads. So far, all have failed "the mission". You may ask why, because many of those civilizations were far more evolved than ours, so what chance do we have?

As I see it, we do have a chance for the following reasons: First, we contain the DNA of previous civilizations within us—the stardust, the vibration, "the remembering" through reincarnations of those who have lived before. And second, we now understand the last piece of the jigsaw—bringing back the balance between male and female: giving and receiving.

As humans, we work with two opposing energies that work together in divine perfection: male and female. Male energy stands for giving; female energy encompasses receiving. These two energies are complete opposites, but to work, create, and grow they must be in balance. The male and female energies are equally powerful. We need both! They need each other! One is not more important than the other. On their own, they cause disruption, ego, pain, and exhaustion. Together, they bring balance, creation, and expansion.

The reason that previous civilizations collapsed was because they chose to continue with only the male energy. We are in danger of doing the exact same thing again, but women are rising up and pushing back. (Please note: Throughout the book, when I speak about "women", I mean all those humans who identify as female. When I speak about "men", I mean all those humans who identify as male.) What we do see, though, is that some protesting feminists forget that we rise as women as equal to men; women/female energy is not more or better or higher than that of men/male energy. Women must rise up and bring back the balance, and men must see and accept this.

## Male Energy

Male energy has been misunderstood for decades. It is seen as the fighting, masculine power that reigns, conquers, and defeats and believed that the only way to receive is through battle, force, and action.

But men are givers, and giving is the male energy. So you must think men's behaviour is correct, because by conquering they can give and provide, a primal thing to do for a man. The thing is, though, that in this closed-consciousness behaviour, the giving can only happen after taking! Taking is not part of the process.

This happened because female energy was singled out and not understood. As a result of closed consciousness, people turned to survival behaviour, one of the lower vibrations, so it grows out of a belief of limitations and control.

There are so many issues with the male ego and the desire to take-take-take that we see on Earth right now. It's because the male energy of giving is becoming so exhausted, caused by imbalance and the inability to receive. When humans feel that they can neither receive nor give anymore, they start to take out of frustration.

Giving and receiving is like a seesaw. One is up, the other is down, then the one is down and the other is up. Up and down, up and down—a beautiful natural play of giving and receiving, tides rolling in and out, life that begins, and life that ends but then reincarnates, like the boomerang that goes out and comes back, the yoyo that goes out and then in, the motion of breath, the woman's cycle, the motion of sex, the cycles of nature, playful, joyful, constant movement.

But if we become stuck, where one is constantly up and the other is constantly down, the joy goes away; the play and the fun. Frustration, anger, and limits are created. This is where the ego, the taking, comes from. The giving is constantly up and the receiving is down. We are not receiving anymore; we only give. But we can't give anymore because the pot is empty. So we start to take, and by taking, there is even more exhaustion, and we destroy creation. There is nothing left. We can't create if we don't receive. We become fully cut-off from source, from our essence. Anxiety, exhaustion, depression, and illnesses take over. This is also creation, but a creation from a lower vibration of loneliness, separation, and feeling of being limited.

## Female Energy

To all who identify as a woman, you will most likely think that we are all about giving? I thought this for an awfully long time. Just like male energy, female energy has also been misunderstood throughout history. It is seen as continuously giving and painfully receiving. Throughout history, receiving has been mostly painful for women, so we have cut it off. For many females, receiving carries a whole load of feelings of guilt, pain, and embarrassment. The female's natural energy of receiving has been replaced by giving. The truth is: Female energy receives and creates!

So here is that missing jigsaw piece! It's in the female energy. Mother Earth is a mirror of us all. Look at the initials. Mother Earth is ME.

Mother Earth is experiencing the exact same thing as the female energy. Like a mirror, she is showing us what we're doing to ourselves. Mother Earth is supposed to receive care and love, and as a result, create food, water, life, enjoyment, physical sensations, and growth for us. Instead, humanity has taken from her, pillaged her. Now she only "gives", and humans take more than she can give. She can't create because she's not given anything to receive. She ends up exhausted. The only thing she can give back is pollution, fire, fear, and death. The female energy is empty.

Women experience an all-time high in fertility problems because they can't give anymore, don't know how to receive anymore, and as a result can't create anymore. Men can't give the sperm anymore as the male energy of giving is no longer there.

I am speaking very generically to make my statement clear. Why has humanity completely lost the true understanding of male and female energy? Because of believing the illusion of limits caused by the physical boundaries we see with our physical eyes.

Everything in a physical experience has a beginning and an end, a first and last, a number, a time limit. Humans are petrified to run out, to not have enough. And yes, in a human experience, we will run out, but only because the man can't give to the woman to receive and create. What happens when that fear comes in? People take. We give royally and constantly when we know we think we won't run out. But most people believe that we will run out of whatever it is. We live inside the illusion of limits, tricked by our human eyes and closed consciousness.

We need to raise human consciousness and vibration and go beyond physical boundaries. This can be done by accepting and practising what is within us all: the balance and constant romantic dance between giving and receiving, the understanding of our unlimited nature and oneness.

Our soul doesn't know such a thing as physical, amount, boundaries, time. That's all an illusion. How do we move away from the illusion of limits and boundaries? How do we bring back the balance between male and female?

The physical crystals were given to us to introduce healing magic and vibrations. They were the first step in waking us up. They connect something physical with energy. In the Aquarian era, we're ascending, away from the physical and towards vibration and limitlessness. We no longer need the physical crystals and instead, to bring back that balance, we must go beyond, returning to our true nature of vibration and limitlessness.

How is this rebalancing of male and female energy connected to ethereal crystals?

Ethereal crystals are not physical, so they are not limited. Ethereal crystals are vibrational, and vibration is unlimited. Ethereal crystals are all about giving. It is the male energy. There is no limit on what we can receive, and as we start to receive that energy in unlimited amounts, we rebalance the beautiful female energy within ourselves. As we receive, we can create new things and give to others, continuing the cycle of giving and receiving.

Our cycle of giving and receiving has just become a whole lot bigger because, as we receive from the unlimited cup of the Universe, there is no limit on what we can continue to give in the physical world. But we must allow ourselves to receive first. We receive from the Universe, which means the Universe gives. The Universe is unlimited; there is no limit on what it receives from itself. The Universe is male and female, everything all at once, always. We are the Universe, we are giving and receiving, male and female all at once. We are the ethereal crystals. The only thing that stands between that and "out of balance" is our limited conscious human mind. All men and women are giving and receiving, all at once.

The male energy gives, the female energy receives, and from that she creates the new. When the new is created, it expands and the female energy gives to others. Now the male also receives from the creation of the female, so he can create and give more and doesn't need to take. She receives again and creates expansion. She shares. He receives from what she created from what he gave her, creates himself, and can now give even more. She receives, creates, and gives. He receives, creates, and gives. She receives, creates, and gives. And so it continues.

There is a beautiful cycle. He is her, she is him, and everything and everyone are one. Giving is receiving; receiving is giving. Total balance—male and female. They become one when worked with and shared as intended. We heal the balance between giving and receiving and raise human consciousness and vibration.

We have now established the following:

- There is only vibration.
- There is only now.
- There is male energy: giving.
- There is female energy: receiving.

- We are all one. Male and female is within us all when it works the way it should, in full connection with the Universe.
- We create a gorgeous dance between male and female, becoming one in creation.
- The ethereal crystals hold all vibration, oneness, and balance now; they are us.
- Human consciousness ascends—vibrations lift.
- Physical experiences transform.
- Humanity and the planet are saved.

## The Destiny of Mother Earth and Humanity

The reason why many people can't ascend is because they are still stuck inside the boundaries of the physical world. When working with ethereal crystals, we allow the ethereal crystals to do the work and, bit by bit, the trust in our true, unlimited, vibrational world comes and the attachment to the physical world goes. When we become detached from what is, creation becomes a fun game of enjoyment, love, happiness, health, and expansion. As a result, human consciousness ascends and vibrations lift.

We can work with ethereal crystals to create new physical crystals in Mother Earth. The formula is as follows:

*Step 1:* Vibration.
*Step 2:* Vibration becomes energy.
*Step 3:* Energy becomes physical form.

When we move the energy of the ethereal crystals (male) into places in Mother Earth (female), she receives and creates new physical crystals and vibrations to give humanity in the following way:

*Step 1:* The vibration of the ethereal crystal.
*Step 2:* The vibration is received by Mother Earth, and Mother Earth creates an energy.
*Step 3:* That energy now takes the physical form of a crystal that can give back to humans and nature.

For example: A high-vibrational physical crystal was removed from a specific place on Earth and now has a low vibration instead of a high one. By placing the new vibration of an ethereal crystal where the physical crystal used to be, we rebalance and heal the vibration in Mother Earth. She has given and now she receives, and she can create a new crystal and give out more positive healing vibrations again.

This is linked to a whole new consciousness of humanity. We will create new physical crystals of a whole new consciousness, lifting "life", "humanity", into a whole new level of existence and consciousness. We'll be creating completely new and different physical outcomes.

At the end of the day, how did physical life come about? It started with a vibration, the consciousness that wanted to be here. We created that together. So we can do that again, but this time with a higher consciousness, a trusting, expanding consciousness of love, health, enjoyment, and abundance.

We can make a huge change. Instead of history repeating, we can create anew in such abundant, beautiful, and conscious ways.

It is important to start working with ethereal crystals in order to make not only the physical world a better place, but also to help grow our collective consciousness. And how do we do that? We do it by becoming aware that the limited physical world we see with our physical eyes is only the materialization of vibration. The physical world we see with our physical eyes, which looks like it is the only thing there is, is actually only a tiny fraction of what life really is.

This realization comes as the result of a growing consciousness in humans that every living experience we have in this physical life can be changed. This change comes not through physical action, not through picking something up and moving it, not through displaying and acting upon big emotions. No, it comes from simply choosing a new vibration.

When we work with ethereal crystals, it is a high vibration harnessed by intention. It is high in divine perfection and alignment with specific goals, depending on the ethereal crystal you choose. By simply choosing certain crystals' vibrations, it will help create a new vibration, which in turn will create a new energy. When the energy is a certain way, the physical world will adapt and change.

We are going to a whole new level: from saving humanity to a whole new human consciousness, which we collectively awaken when we see that we are the creators of our own lives. We also get to see how I am you and you are me. I create anew, I give, and by so doing, you can receive; and by receiving, your vibration will change, and you can create anew and give; and so on and on. What you do is for me. What I do is for you. By changing that vibration, I heal that which is in me and you.

By itself, the physical world is limited until the human's mind remembers its limitlessness. The giving needs the receiving to create. The receiving needs the giving to create. The physical world needs the energetic world. And that becomes a beautiful circle of life, of creation, positive change, healing, and transformation. Ethereal crystals have always been there, but we were too attached to the physical world to see them. Now we're ready, as we collectively ascend.

The meditation in Part Three of this book, "Communicating with and Embodying the Wisdom of Ethereal Crystals", will help you connect with this new consciousness, this new vibration, this healing of "giving and receiving". You can read the meditation while visualizing and feeling what I describe or record it and connect that way.

# 5

# Control versus Trust

## Appreciating the Magic of Trust

As humans have become so attached to the physical world, they have picked up the habit of controlling the physical world by using only physical action. They think that the only way things can get done is by using physical action. Nothing could be further from the truth.

The only time we need to physically act is when the action is in alignment with the new vibration, but most human actions reflect a desperate attempt to control things.

There are two different types of control: one that does not support our wellbeing and the other that does.

The first arises from fear and lack of trust and leads to depression, anxiety, sickness, and unimaginable loss of control. The more you try to control things, the less control you seemingly have, so you keep trying to control things even more, and so it continues in a vicious circle.

We also try to control things by placing unrealistic expectations on something or someone we think will be good for us. Whenever you place expectations on others, you're blocking the flow of your highest good by trying to control outcomes. So, when you see something you'd love to have in your life, instead of overloading it with the weight of your expectations, just say, "Yes, please!" The Universe will then bring you what you are asking for, or even better. You can trust that.

You only have to read history books, or look at certain countries today, to see how humans have not felt safe, which has led them to live in constant fight-or-flight mode, and this continues even today. The feeling of being physically unsafe is the root cause of people desperately trying to control life. In that state, their sole focus is on physical actions, not changing the vibration underlying the feeling.

The second type of control is what we're aiming for here. It is the type of control where you know with full confidence where you want to be and what you want. You feel it, believe it, and even when you are filled with doubt, you still know that it's yours (or something better), because you trust in the unknown and higher power and thus, have total control. As a result, what you want to create in your physical world is exactly what will be boomeranged back to you, or better. This is positive control.

Trust is a strong vibration. When you trust, you become one with all that is. All that is has your highest good and purpose in it, often a thousand times more glorious than you could have ever imagined. Being aware is a major part of the healing process. The more you try to control, the more you block any process. Acknowledge it, and let it go. Take a deep breath.

Once we let go, we're in control—magnificent positive control. We don't have to force, because fear is not involved. We know that all is perfect. We are the creators, and we create with vibration. To receive, we need to trust. When we fear rejection or abandonment, we're not trusting. When there's no trust, there's no flow, and we can't receive. A trusting vibration is high and open, a superhighway where travel is smooth and has no speed limit so you reach your destination quickly and without a hitch. A controlling vibration is low and feels like navigating a complex obstacle course.

My husband is an absolute star in controlling life through trust. A few years ago, we lived comfortably in our beautiful home in Essex in the UK, and I loved my house, my friends, and my life. Things weren't perfect, and cracks were starting to appear, but I hung on tight to our perfect location and life there, and every day, I focused on putting out the vibration that represented my perfect life so the cracks would smooth out.

One day, my husband came home and said, "What if we moved to Ireland?"

My first thought was *No way! I love it here, and I'm creating my perfect life here!* I couldn't see how his idea was part of my creation and was set against it. When our house didn't sell immediately, I thought it wasn't meant to be, and my initial rebellion turned into trust. I had been putting my "perfect vibe" out there, so now I needed to trust that the physical results might be different than what I was expecting.

I kept creating without thinking of the physical outcome of where, how, and who. I released the attachment to the town and people where we lived, and I flowed. This way I removed all obstacles on the path, and I was driving on my metaphorical German superhighway.

Not long after that, we had an offer on the house, my husband went to Ireland to look for a new house, and on one of the last days of his search, our dream property came on the market. Thanks to moving, our lives and the kids' lives transformed in more and bigger ways than we could have ever thought possible. I created this move by creating the right vibration I wanted in my life and trusted that the Universe knew exactly where to guide me to achieve that. The Universe responds to vibration because that's what it is and that's what we are: vibration!

Trust is:

1  No attachment to specific outcomes
2  Continuously uplifting your vibration
3  Creating with your true essence = divinely high vibrations and trust

It works the same way with ethereal crystals. Unlike physical crystals, we can't see ethereal crystals, which can cause a lot of doubt; we just know why we call them in and what we want as a result. Still, we can't "see" them. This is where trust comes in—trusting the Universe, trusting the power of the Self, trusting your connection to all that is.

That is one powerful way of controlling. By just focusing on a particular ethereal crystal, we can change, heal, create, and transform. Wow! Trusting, accepting, and receiving are a big part of the message of the ethereal crystals.

The opposite of trust is rejection. Letting go of rejection means accepting yourself. When you are not experiencing flow, wealth, health, and love in your life, it means you are rejecting it within yourself. Letting go of rejection means accepting yourself. When you accept yourself, you come into full alignment with your truth: health, wealth, happiness, love, and abundance.

Accepting yourself can be difficult if you have never been shown the way to do that. Working with ethereal crystals offers a perfect means to get there. Trust in them. Trust in their vibration. Trust in their magic. Bit by bit, accept that you *are* the ethereal crystals, you *are* a part of that high vibration. Accept that you are all that is, in divine perfection.

Here's a beautiful exercise I channelled. You can do this to work on the process of accepting yourself and to trust your flow.

## Exercise

Place your hands on your breasts—let the word "nurturing" circle and vibrate in your chest—nurturing yourself. Flow your hands down onto your belly, one hand on top of the other. Keep your attention on your womb/belly. Let the word "nurturing" create, circle, and vibrate. You are the creator of your whole existence. Breathe into it. Feel it. Send out that vibration. Slide your left hand down your left leg and your right hand down your right leg. Push the vibration down into your earthly consciousness. Circle your hands up onto your head, stroking your hair down your ears and neck, back onto your breasts. Repeat this cycle five times.

# Positive Intention
# and Free Will

## Respecting the Power of Intention
## and Others' Free Will

Ethereal crystals can only be placed and work when the intention is pure and from the heart; in other words, when the intention is positive. Always remind yourself, no matter how good your intentions, the outcome is always what will be best for them.

Here we are again with trust! Free will to accept or not is always part of the human equation.

My brother-in-law, aged just 41 years old, was extremely ill in hospital in Spain. My husband rushed to be with him, while I stayed at home and sent him healing vibrations. Although I did this with the best of intentions and love, almost immediately after "sending" out the healing vibrations, they came straight back to me with the message: "It is my time. Thank you, but don't."

I accepted his message. A few hours later, before my husband had even reached Spain, I received a phone call to say that he had passed away. The vibrations had arrived and would have helped him, but he decided not to accept.

I believe in karma; that is, what you send out comes back to you. Use ethereal crystals and intentions with purity of heart and intention, love, and trust. Positive intention paired with ethereal crystals always works, but humans have the free will to accept or decline their help.

Another beautiful story was when I was on the Neonatal Intensive Care Unit. I felt this heavy energy around a baby boy lying there. He had been distressed during birth and had defecated in the water and started breathing it in while still in the womb. This had damaged his lungs and potentially also his brain. The baby boy was intubated and had severe problems.

I asked the Universe, "Am I allowed to heal without someone's permission?" The answer was "You can only do good with healing from the heart, which you are doing. Heal, and then it is up to them to receive or reject it. That is the free will of human beings."

# Visualization

## The Power of Using Your Imagination

Visualization can play a key role in the creation process; or rather, it can make the process easier! Visualization helps us believe that healing and change are occurring. Even though we must believe it to see it, we all like to see to believe, don't we?

This is where visualization comes in. Visualization is simply imagining your desired outcome with the right emotion attached to it. Just like riding a bike, you can improve by practising. Look around you a bit less, and start visualizing a bit more.

We work with ethereal crystals by visualizing each crystal's gorgeous energy using whatever colours and shapes come to you. This helps guide the vibration of the ethereal crystal to where you want it. You see it in your mind's eye. You feel it in every fibre of your body, then *boom*, it settles where needed and does its work, then you let go.

You can also visualize the wished-for outcome and see the relationship, body part, business, and emotions transform right after guiding the ethereal crystal where needed. Then you let go and trust. It is done.

You can visually focus on the beautiful photographs in this book, and use them to guide you and visualize their vibration. Here are some easy exercises you can do regularly to improve your visualization skills.

## Exercises

Take an object (e.g., a book, a cup, a dress, a pretty box), and stare at the object. Look at every detail, and take it all in. When you feel ready, close your eyes and recall the object you just observed. Recall every little detail, and see it all in your mind. Imagine short scenes with your eyes closed. Once you get better at this, imagine short scenes with your eyes open. As you get better, your imagined scenes can get longer.

Your third eye, the seat of "seeing", is located between your eyebrows on your forehead. You can help open it by staring into the distance. Meditate while you hold your full attention on your third eye. Imagine an eye, and see what happens. Allow images to come and go.

It is all about visualization, positive intention, trust, and once done, letting go and knowing that change has taken place. You must let go and trust. Remember the chapter when I spoke about control? You will have control when you trust that the Universe is taking control for the highest good and purpose of everything and everyone involved, now and always, and so it is.

The visualizing part can help create the trust part, as very often, we need to "see" to believe. Well, visualize it yourself, feel how that is what you want to realize and then trust that it is working.

We are vibration, and vibration never disappears. It was here then, is here now, and will be here forever. It is ever changing, depending on how we mould it. Neither time nor space exist. Vibration is here now, and its effects ripple in all directions of time and space, everyone involved.

# 8

# Ethereal Crystals
## Understanding How Ethereal Crystals Work

In their essence, ethereal crystals represent the energy of all crystals— their consciousness in all directions of time and space, all dimensions, all civilizations, and the Universe. They are pure vibration.

We are a part of that, too. Thus, when we connect with ethereal crystals, it is a remembering, a reconnecting with ourselves and our unlimited nature.

Humans experience life as a world of physical manifestations so we like to give things names. Working with ethereal crystals is an in-between step to becoming, to reconnecting with oneness. It is a bridge to fully letting go of the illusion of separation in a conscious way. We are everything the ethereal crystals give us. We are all that already. The ethereal crystals have come to remind us of all that.

## What Are Ethereal Crystals?

The meaning of ethereal crystals can be described in just one word. That one word is their lesson, message, and meaning: Vibration.

When creating with ethereal crystals, you only need one person to know that everything is perfect health, happiness, love, and abundance. By placing the energy of crystals where needed, it reminds the other person, even subconsciously, that they are one, and that spark creates immediate healing on whatever level needed and accepted.

Ethereal crystals represent, remind us of, and bring, all that is: perfect health, happiness, love, abundance. By bringing ethereal crystals into human consciousness, we are healing humanity. We are reconnecting with the collective consciousness. We are restoring the balance between male and female. We become aware of the illusion created by physical boundaries.

The following is a more technical explanation of what ethereal crystals are and how they work.

When we work with ethereal crystals, the Universe directly gives us the strength and power of the crystal, which we then place simply by intention. Ethereal crystals are some four hundred times stronger (and so much more) than those found on Earth, because they are pure and come directly from the Universe. Human tissue manifests from vibrations, and ethereal crystals are powerful vibrations.

Where there are blockages, pain, or disease, the vibration of wherever the problem is has changed. When we place an ethereal crystal on the body, its vibration will influence the changed frequencies in the body and bring it back into balance. The body will react to the vibration of the ethereal crystal. Ethereal crystals also have an incredible influence on emotional and psychological health. It is important to choose the right ethereal crystal, or several in combination. It is possible to capture the vibrations of ethereal crystals purely by intention.

Here are some benefits of using ethereal crystals for healing and creation:

- The healing energy is always in its full form and strength.
- You don't need to look after the crystal.
- The crystal is always the right one for you, unlike a physical crystal, which requires you to find the right one for it to work.
- You can use ethereal crystals to offer healing and protection or transmit energy to someone, even when you're on the other side of the world.
- Once the energy of the crystal is placed, it fades all by itself when no longer needed. Unlike physical crystals, ethereal crystals cannot be dislodged by movement or activity. You can place them in or on everything and everyone, simply by positive strong intention.

- You can make gem elixirs in seconds.
- You can also cleanse and strengthen a physical crystal by skilfully working with ethereal crystals.

Life is in the mind. We use our intention to go to the front door when we want to leave the house. We use our intention to take a drink when we're thirsty. It is all intention. Even when you're not doing anything, it still is an intention. Everything in life starts with an intention. This is what sparks and attracts the vibration.

Healing and creating with ethereal crystals works the exact same way: by intention. Don't let your current programmed vibration make you think you can't change! You continue because it is often a deep well of emotion after emotion, blockage and belief after blockage and belief. If you continue, you will create a new body, mind, emotions, and life.

As noted earlier, we experience negative emotions because we identify with what we are seeing with our physical eyes. But what we are seeing with our physical eyes is simply a reflection of our vibration.

When you use your intention to change a negative emotion using the power of ethereal crystals, you are activating a new consciousness. This higher consciousness allows you to regain your power of creation, positive control, knowing, and trust. As you allow the ethereal crystal vibration into your life, emotions will be lifted, and as a result, the illusion you create becomes positive instead of negative.

As long as you are living the human experience, what you experience will be an illusion. But part of playing the game is to realize that you are the creator, you are every level of vibration and creation all at once. You can choose the vibration. The ethereal crystals have come to remind you of that and to help create once more.

There are four steps in the creation process:

1 **Accountability:** This means that you, and only you, can create your transformation. You can help others with your knowledge when they are being accountable and come to you for guidance and support. As an individual with free will, you must take the responsibility for change.

2 **Awareness:** Become aware of your patterns, your beliefs, your aches and pains, and the messages behind them. Listen to your body. See the environment you've attracted. You must be aware of all that and know that you created it, before you can change it. You can't know what you love if you can't see and feel what you don't.

3 **Transform:** Work with ethereal crystals to create new vibrations.

4 **Persist:** The higher your consciousness goes, the faster the changes and creations will happen, often immediately. Until then, remember that everything new is a process. It is as if you're in a rehabilitation centre. Your body and mind have gone through hell, but now you're starting again and being supported every step of the way. The rehab techniques can be found in this book. Every day, you practise, read, learn, practise some more, read, learn. You fall, doubt, but get up again. This is a real awakening. And one day, you will wake up and realize that so much has changed and you've transformed.

# Working with Ethereal Crystals

## Connecting, Communicating, and Placing Ethereal Crystals where Needed

Place your chosen ethereal crystals by pointing with your finger (or with your mind only) to the place where the crystal is needed and saying the crystal's name, either out loud or silently in your mind; for example: "Place rose quartz in the heart." The crystal(s) will then be placed instantly.

Ethereal crystals can be placed wherever needed, including in:

- Organs
- The body
- Buildings (or around them)
- Situations
- Past lives
- Animals
- Plants
- Water
- Energies
- Vibrations
- Food
- Connections between people
- Absolutely anything

There are no distance restrictions with this healing method. It works instantly, even on someone or in places on the other side of the world, even other planets or galaxies. You ask for the vibration of the crystal, and the Universe gives it instantly. As noted, neither time nor space exist; everything happens in the here and now.

After placing the crystals, other healing methods can be performed or you can just let the ethereal crystals do their work. Even though it is unnecessary, you can always remove the ethereal crystal by thinking or saying, "Remove [name of the crystal]."

## How Do They Work?

Ethereal crystals come straight from the Universe, so they vibrate in a vibrant, strong, powerful, perfect, and divine way. The body part, room, or connection that needs the ethereal crystal vibrates in a completely different way, which may make the room uncomfortable, the organ malfunction, the blood clot, relationships difficult, and so on. By placing the high vibration of the ethereal crystal where needed, it will influence the lower vibration to speed up, lift in its vibration, and flow divinely. As a result, the room may feel comfortable again, the organ become healthy and work perfectly, the blood flow easily, relationships improve, negative feelings disappear, and so on.

## My Revelation

The first time I worked with ethereal crystals was a revelation. I was doing a healing session with a client and gave her a specific crystal to hold while I was working on an issue to help move things along.

The client kept the crystals in her hands, even when the next one was added, and I felt that this lady needed these crystals with her longer, but that was not possible once the session was finished.

As I was thinking about this, my spirit guides told me to imagine placing the crystals into the heart of my client so they could keep working after she went home, which I proceeded to do. I felt the extraordinary strength of the healing power as I placed the "imagined crystals" in her heart, and because of this, I have worked this way ever since.

I am excited about the potential of working with ethereal crystals because it makes healing easy and open to everyone. Many people don't have the time to sit down and clear crystals or take the time to place them or recharge them. Working with ethereal crystals offers instant healing and makes even the most rare and expensive crystals available to you. You don't have to find the right one, you don't need to get your purse out; you simply ask for it, and it is there. How fantastic is that?

## When Can I Start Working with Ethereal Crystals?

After my fabulous, guided moment, I was so excited. I told a close friend of mine about what had just happened, and she decided to give me an attunement to work with ethereal crystals.

It was a lovely experience, and I was incredibly grateful to her, so I went ahead with it. But I had already worked with the ethereal crystals, so why did I need an attunement?

The short answer is: You don't.

Of course, everyone needs to figure that out for themselves. If you feel better having an attunement, find someone who can give you one, but just know that you don't need one to work with ethereal crystals. Every one of us is connected to all the people, all the places, and all the animals on this planet. We are all one with and part of the universe where the ethereal crystals have their home. When the intention is good and is given with love, this is all that's needed. Go ahead—heal, create, and transform your life and that of others with ethereal crystals.

# Medical versus Energy Healing

## The Magical Cooperation between Medical and Energy Healing

Based on everything I've spoken about so far, we can conclude the following:

- Everything physical exists because of vibration, so changing vibration = transforming life.
- There is only the now.
- To expand, male and female energies need to dance in perfect harmony with one another: giving, receiving, creating; giving, receiving, creating.
- By doing this, we create balance and allow consciousness and vibration to ascend.

Ethereal crystals help change the vibration, creating improved relationships, healthy businesses, money flow, happiness, and whatever else you want to create.

*Vibration > creates energy > determines the physical outcome*

Let's look at the following statement: "Physically, some things are a lot harder to heal than others." It is one thing to believe we can instantly manifest things we desire and heal small physical ailments; it is another thing to believe we can instantly heal "serious" illnesses.

I place "serious" in quotation marks because in truth, nothing is too big or too small to heal. That's just another illusion. I do believe that humanity is not strong enough yet, collectively, to heal certain physical issues instantly. We are still very attached to the illusion of time; as explained earlier, it is a process. What can happen, though, is that medical and energy healing can collaborate until our vibration is high enough and we no longer need medical healing. When that time comes, illness will no longer exist, so we won't need medical healing, anyway. Until then, let's work with both for the best outcomes.

When my daughter was born just 24 weeks into my pregnancy, I was faced with this big question of medical versus energy healing. I had been studying and working within the field of energy healing for many years at that point, and this was a real moment of truth. I was forced to face what I was sharing with the world, put it under the loop, and fully integrate it into my being: "We can heal and create anything."

And then the Universe brought me my 1lb baby.

There she was, my tiny 500-gram baby. "Who am I to do this work? Who am I to heal her?" These were two questions that came up.

Her eyes were still fused shut, her brain hadn't unfolded yet, her skin was sticky red, her lungs were damaged, and she couldn't breathe on her own. She had a severe streptococcus A infection, and so did I. When she was born, her body was so fragile she was covered in bruises. This meant that there could be bleeding inside her body.

Right after she was born, I collapsed. I was at the bottom of the barrel. The nurses had to carry me to bed. *How on earth am I supposed to deal with this?* I thought.

The room was heaving with medical practitioners and curious people, but I completely surrendered. It was in that moment, when I had let go of all resistance, that I was suddenly surrounded by the most peaceful vibration I have ever experienced. It was out of this world. If I could, I would have bottled it to share with you.

It was Source energy—the highest, deepest peace, the perfect everything. I knew in that moment that, even though nothing was okay in my physical world, everything was in fact okay; because that feeling

I was surrounded by was our Source—yours, mine, and my baby's. I started doing the work immediately.

Physically, my baby's body was not ready to live. We needed the collaboration of medical and vibrational healing. We worked on the physical level with traditional medicine and on the vibrational level with energy healing.

That was when the true miracles took place. The only way she could get oxygen into her lungs was via intubation. At that moment, she needed that physical intervention. The vibrational change to create a perfect physical outcome was where my work came in.

Let's not forget that it was my vibration that had brought us there. I say that with the greatest respect and warmth towards myself, but I also know that that was true. You create your own reality on absolutely every level. The moment you take full responsibility for that, true transformation can take place.

My husband was away a lot for work. I felt abandoned. My father left my mother when I was five. He left me. That vibration was still reverberating for me. My mother never spoke up against my father. Men were dominant communicators in my family line. I couldn't say to my husband how I was feeling.

I developed a streptococcus A infection. It started in my throat. I couldn't say what I was feeling. It affected my womb, the epicentre of all emotions. I was pregnant, so it affected my pregnancy. My vibration had brought me to that moment.

It suddenly all made sense, and I deep-dived into what I know best: changing vibration to transform life. The doctors said, only one or two babies out of ten, born as prematurely as my daughter, would live to be perfectly healthy.

A beautiful example of this: Because my daughter was born extremely premature, her ductus arteriosus, a blood vessel connecting the fetal pulmonary artery to the heart aorta allowing oxygenated blood to provide nutrition in the womb, did not close after birth. That normally happens right away, when a newborn takes its first breath, but it didn't happen with her. The doctor gave her medicine to assist, so I thought, *Okay, they are doing their thing, and I will work on it vibrationally.*

I worked on the vibrational levels of her heart and lungs, her ductus, and everything that needed to be physically fixed. If not, she would have needed an operation. The result was that after just one dose of the medicine and my vibrational work, her ductus closed. The doctors couldn't believe it, as she was born not just premature but extremely premature. This was very rare.

We are multidimensional beings. The body reacts to our vibration. The body is the way it is because of the vibration. We are physically here, but as I have noted, it is the vibration that creates that physical world. Until we make a collective return to the consciousness that our natural state is perfect health, love, and abundance, we need to collaborate with the medical world for healing as and when needed. The more we collaborate, the more our collective consciousness and vibration can shift and the less illness there will be, allowing a return to a physical life in our natural state of perfect health.

Because of my daughter's extremely premature birth, the doctors said that she would have chronic lung disease. They said that there was nothing they could do about it. They saw it as "the result" of and "the reaction" to her extreme premature birth, something she would have to carry her whole life.

That went in one ear and out the other, as I refused to take on that belief, already knowing that her natural state is perfect health. They clearly didn't understand how creation really works, so I did something about it.

I worked deeply on the vibrational level of her lungs. The lungs are linked to the heart chakra, so I also worked on her heart energy. I imagined her beautiful lungs. I would clean them out completely in my imagination, as there were a lot of dead alveoli. I imagined seeing them healthy and green (the colour of healing). I placed the vibration of the ethereal crystals in her lungs, in her heart chakra, and placed new vibrations on her connection with me. As she was my baby, chalcedony strengthens the bond between mother and child. I placed chalcedony in the soles of her feet to heal emotions. The lungs stand for the breathing in of joy. I placed chalcedony in her lungs.

Here is the result: She went to nursery when she was just two years old. She has never had any more colds or coughs than any of my other children; she might even have had fewer! She definitely never has had any issues with chronic lung disease, none whatsoever.

There will come a day when there are no negative vibrations, no more karma to solve, only positivity, and you won't need medical healing anymore because you will be in full alignment with your true self again, with Source—love, happiness, perfect health, and abundance. It is important we wake up to that.

Working with ethereal crystals is a part of the return to our natural state, of who we are. Many people will be left behind because they are stuck in the physical cycle, the karmic cycle, the negativity. But because you are starting to combine medical and vibrational healing, you're moving forward towards a point where you don't need medical healing anymore. You'll be back in full alignment, and you won't even get sick. That's how you can help others do the same. That's how we raise vibration and rise together.

It bears repeating: In essence, what we truly are is perfect health. Our natural state is perfect health, perfect love, perfect happiness, perfect abundance. That is our true essence. Anything else is an illusion.

Many people get sick, receive medical treatment, and get sick again. They live a life believing in limitations. They believe the body and mind have limits. I really hope you now understand that the truth is the exact opposite.

Until the vibration has been changed, the physical issues, emotional pain, bad relationships, and money issues will keep coming back. Vibrational change is the root of all transformation.

# Shapes and Ethereal Crystals
## Enhancing Results with Crystalline Shapes

A crystalline shape is a vibrational shape held together in an ordered arrangement of ethereal crystals. Because each ethereal crystal within the crystalline shape has its own vibration, placing them together magnifies the overall vibration and offers the highest order of action.

There are two different ways to create ethereal crystalline shapes:

- **Imagination:** Use your imagination to create the crystalline shape, and then use your intention to add ethereal crystals to the shape.
- **Intention:** Say the name of the shape and the ethereal crystals. For example: "I place a Pyramid of ruby, tourmaline, and citrine above the head." You already know what you want to achieve when asking for it, so trust the Universe to create the divinely perfect pyramid and organization of the vibrations.

## Horizontal Line

A Horizontal line of ethereal crystals will support the purging of old ideas, beliefs, and programming.

## Circle

The Circle is linked to the celestial plane. It is the strongest shape in nature, as vibration is distributed equally all the way around. The Circle stands for growth and expansion and brings in life force and energy. Place nine ethereal crystals in a Circle for help with:

- Personal will
- Firm direction linked to the soul's will
- Remembering the soul's plan
- Breathing life into your creation
- Creating
- Becoming pregnant
- Creating passion
- Shifting from old to new
- Being reborn
- Going beyond physical boundaries

## Concentric Circles

A Concentric Circle shape is used for success and abundance. In the middle of the home, place one main ethereal crystal, then seven ethereal crystals spread around the first crystal in a circle (seven crystals are used as the number seven stands for movement). Around that first circle, place another seven of the same ethereal crystals, then do the same in another circle of seven crystals around the second to really push the energy into the house. The energy vibrates outward like tree rings on a tree trunk or a pebble thrown into a pond, getting bigger as they radiate outwards. Use a Concentric Circle for issues to do with:

- Life and death
- Bringing our babies to us
- Helping release the spirits of people who have crossed over
- Physical healing
- Grounding
- Raising vibrations
- Creating abundance

## Spiral

Place your chosen ethereal crystals in a Spiral shape along the energy centres known as the chakras, from the feet to the top of the head, to bring alignment between mind and body.

## Tornado

To cleanse your house or any other building, use the Tornado of diamond energy shape. Have it go from corner to corner and cleanse the whole room or building, then descend into Mother Earth via the pipes in one or all corners of the building.

## Triangle

The Triangle shape is used to cleanse or empower, depending on whether the point is pointing up or down.

Have the point pointing down:

- For breaking addiction
- To cleanse and remove "sickness" vibrations after illness

Have the triangle pointing up:

- To build something up, such as muscle strength or confidence
- To recover from illness

To heal the heart space and to remember all that is—love—meditate in the following way: Place a single ethereal crystal green amethyst in the heart, and place the shape of a Triangle around it. Then imagine sitting inside a big Triangle shape. Place a purple amethyst in the crown chakra (on the top of the head) where the tip of the triangle is, and place two more purple amethysts on the other two corners of the triangle.

## Three-Sided Pyramid

The Pyramid crystalline shape helps you grow and reach a higher state of being, enter a whole new level of healing, and start a new story.

A Pyramid shape is perfect when seeking:

- Rejuvenation
- Healing in the deepest cells
- Healing of the DNA
- Healing in all directions of time and space

Place Pyramid shapes in the body. One up, one down, with bases attached to one another, a powerful configuration because the adjoining bases represent the physical world. The top triangle brings down the giving energy; the bottom point, the receiving. This is a true dynamic force of creation, actively and consciously creating and bringing to life the ancient principle of "As above, so below; as within, so without" in physical form.

Use the four-sided Pyramid to treat muscular and bone issues.

## Four-Sided Pyramid

Imagine a Four-Sided Pyramid shape with the ethereal crystals of your choice to:

- Create a path towards enlightenment
- Remember that everything is possible

## Square

The shape of earthly world protection and grounding, the Square shape can support grounding and healing when suffering from:

- Feeling physically unstable on the feet
- Headaches
- Light-headedness
- Illnesses that make people try to run away from their thoughts—dementia, coma, stroke, and so on.
- Insecurity
- Doubt

The Square shape also offers support for:

- Removing toxins, so that Mother Earth can transmute them.
- Making you feel safe and healing fears around physical safety.
- Grounding your spiritual awakening when used during meditation.
- Helping bring new awakening into your consciousness.
- Looking for a new home, the best town to live in.

# Hexagon

Work with the Hexagon shape when you're looking for:

- A team
- A community
- To create together in balance

The Hexagon has six sides. The number six stands for:

- Making decisions
- Being strong individually but working in a divinely perfect way in a team.
- Equality
- Strength

The Hexagon shape is a powerful one to use when creating a team/community because pressure is divided equally, so it stands for strong and long-lasting relationships. In traditional Chinese literature, the Hexagon stands for North, West, East, South, Heaven, and Earth—Completeness.

## Octagon

When creating an Octagon shape, work with the ethereal crystal of fluorite as an ascension tool. Work with this shape:

- To focus
- To be all-encompassing
- To lead

Fluorite stands for rebirth, and the eight-sided Octagon shape stands for realignment. Place fluorite crystals in an Octagon shape around a person, and one in the pelvis to heal blood diseases.

This shape and ethereal crystal can be a big support in the transition from the earthly plane of lower vibrations to the celestial plane of higher vibrations, a return to our natural state of perfect health, love, happiness, and abundance.

## Star Grid

We place a Star Grid in Mother Earth for:

- Intergalactic healing
- Connection with other planets

On the physical, emotional, etheric, spiritual, and causal level, this is a very deep healing allowing you to cleanse and renew. This will heal:

- Detrimental entities
- Negative thought forms
- Negativity
- Soul wound healing in all directions of time and space and everyone involved.

## Numbers

You can also place ethereal crystals in a Number shape. Use the different numbers for help with:

**Number 1:** A new beginning and good communication.

**Number 2:** Dealing with emotions and reaching a deeper connection with intuition.

**Number 3:** Becoming a parent, inviting something new into life, and creating pure physical enjoyment.

**Number 4:** Becoming a boss, leadership, strength, grounding, success, and money.

**Number 5:** Receiving wisdom, guidance, mentorship, and clarity.

**Number 6:** Being presented with choices and receiving support in decision-making and healing deep emotions.

**Number 7:** Creating movement and letting go of what weighs too heavy.

**Number 8:** Rebalancing, and to be, create, and act appropriately.

**Number 9:** Standing in your power without being influenced by others, and shining and being seen.

**Number 10:** Receiving a fast turnaround and positive changes.

# Seeing Crystal Vibrations with the Naked Eye

## The Biofield Imaging Images

Unfortunately, it is impossible to share images of the actual ethereal crystals, as they are a vibration/energy from a different dimension. The colours and vibrations of ethereal crystals are a thousand times higher and more vibrant than those of physical crystals. Subsequently, we are unable to compare the two in a visual way.

I wanted to share photographs of physical crystals with you, as they are beautiful, physical proof of how everything vibrates. These crystals were photographed with a normal camera and processed by Biofield Imaging software. (www.biofieldimaging.com)

Certain crystals appear more vitalizing (yellow), while others appear as a mixture of balance (green) and higher frequency (orange/gold). I cannot emphasize enough that ethereal crystals are divinely perfect and contain the highest light and colours. They are matched perfectly for what each person needs, as they are beyond this physical world.

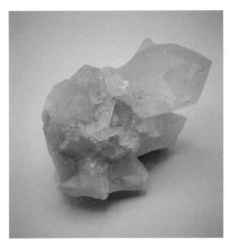
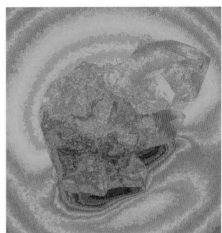

Clear Quartz

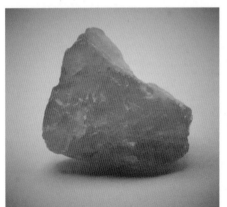
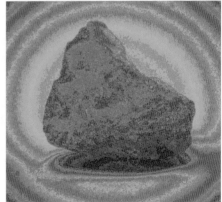

Rose Quartz

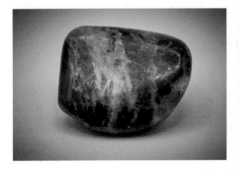
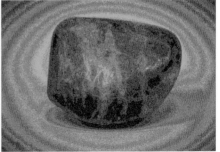

Sodalite

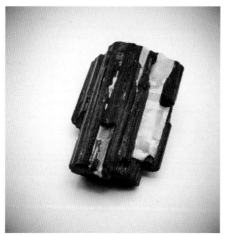 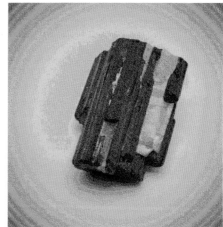

Tourmaline

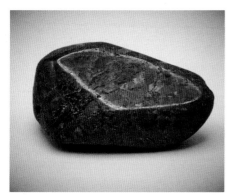 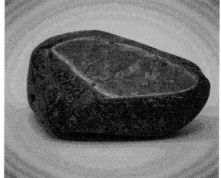

Unakite

# Part Two

# 33 Ethereal Crystals and Their Healing Powers

# 33 Ethereal Crystals
## Healing Powers
## and Messages

Descriptions of each crystal are accompanied by a photograph of the physical crystal. I have empowered each photograph of the physical crystal with its ethereal crystal counterpart, which means that the photographs in this book are highly vibrational. You can work with them by connecting with them. Breathe in their healing and creative powers while setting your intention about why you are tuning in. Or you can just look at or simply sit in front of the image and allow its energy to reach you vibrationally.

Here is a quick reminder of how to use the images:

1  Set your intention. Say out loud or in your mind what it is that you want to manifest or transform.

2  If you would like to work with a specific coloured crystal, choose your colour crystal and also set that intention.

3  Thank the crystal for now bringing its vibration to where it is needed.

4  Close your eyes and breathe as you allow the vibration of the image to do its work.

# Agate

*Pharmacy*

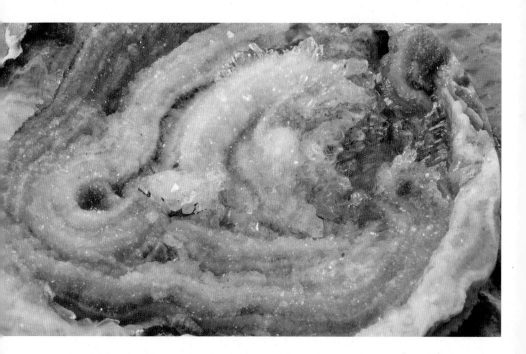

J ust like the physical crystal, agate ethereal crystal can be channelled in many different colours. Depending on your need, you can choose a different colour. Depending on the chosen colour, the energy will be different. If this sounds confusing, don't worry at all about the colour, and just continue to focus on the intention of why you're calling in the vibration of the ethereal crystal. The Universe always knows which one is best, as it responds to the vibration of your intent.

Agate is an ethereal crystal that should not be missed, as it has fabulous healing power—truly a one-crystal-heals-all energy. When in doubt as to which ethereal crystal to use, go for agate. This is also a gorgeous energy for children. Agate energy is a natural painkiller and calms and protects against influences when feeling depressed and suffering from phobias.

When pregnant and during delivery, orange agate is the perfect energy to place around you. Agate protects mother and child during pregnancy, makes a heavy delivery lighter, helps reduce pain and makes pain bearable, and helps heal (potential) infections.

When people feel angry, there is always an underlying emotion of hopelessness linked to the anger. Place the energy of yellow agate in the solar plexus to calm anger and heal hopelessness, so that the vibration changes and the reason behind the hopelessness can be released. When those roots have been removed, the anger can't be manifested. Fever and high blood pressure represent anger.

When struggling with physical issues such as these, place the energy of agate in the solar plexus. The solar plexus is situated where the stomach is. Say, "Place yellow agate in the solar plexus."

Similar to a painkiller in traditional medicine, we can use agate energy in vibrational healing. When suffering from colds, tinnitus, head colds, place the blue agate ethereal crystal where needed.

Purple agate energy can be channelled to heal dizziness. Use your intention to place this vibration in your head, and visualize gorgeous purple energy filling the space and vibrating slowly outside the boundaries of your cranium.

White agate energy will help increase mental acuity, give insights, and support inner development. You can envelop your body and head with this ethereal crystal and/or place it by intention in your head (for dizziness) or mind (for insights and inner development).

# Amber

## *Witches' Fire*

Amber ethereal crystal is a powerful energy that carries many purposes. The amber energy is here for all those witches who were burned at the stake and forcefully removed from life for understanding vibration. Amber energy is here to make the witches remember. You can see the amber in your mind's eye as a warm orange light. The orange represents fire. When we keep burning our own fire, it can never be burned by others, no matter what.

Amber has a big spiritual impact and has been associated with magic for years. It is a protective stone for Wiccans and shamans. It carries the knowledge and whispers of our Wiccan ancestors. Meditating on this beautiful energy can help you connect with those ancestors and their knowledge.

Amber is also a sensual, magnetic energy that attracts love. You only have to look at fire to understand this. Love and sensuality are a beautiful, warm fire. Connect with this energy, surround yourself with it, in order to change your vibration so you can heal and enter the level of the perfect fire to attract love and positive passion into your life.

It is the perfect energy to work with to protect against negative influences and black magic. Place that energy by intention where the protection is needed. Your gut feeling will always know where that is, so don't doubt it! Say: "Place amber around/in/on [insert place]" accompanied by the intention of what you want to create.

When there is a struggle with fear, depression, phobias, fatigue, or a weak immune system, use strong intention as you place the energy of amber around the person who is suffering, so that they can remember their fire, their fight, and their passion.

If someone is struggling with arthritis, osteoarthritis, or rheumatism, place the energy of amber in their joints accompanied by the intention of your desired result. If the disease presents in other places, such as the eyes, the lungs, the skin, or the heart, place the amber energy there. In this way, you bring fire energy back into the heart, the lungs, the skin, the joints so that the person can love, breathe, enjoy, and move freely through life.

To heal varicose veins, liver problems, and hay fever, work with the energy of amber to balance fire. These physical manifestations happen when someone feels angry about wanting and desiring passion in their lives.

Amber energy can be placed in the gums when the teeth of small children push through or placed in the gums when someone is suffering from gum inflammation or an abscess.

When people suffer from acute skin rash or psoriasis, the vibration is one of not feeling safe in one's own skin. They feel unloved, flaky, too

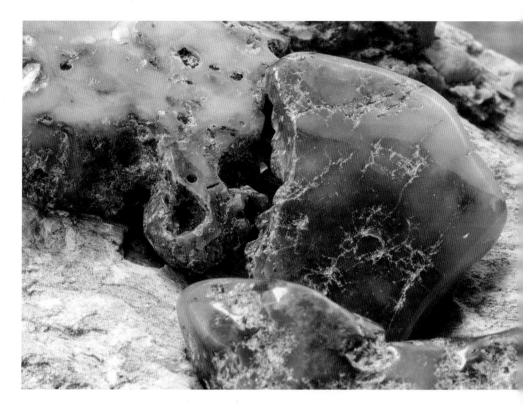

hard, too hurt, too sensitive. Placing the energy of amber on the rash can help heal that vibration. Also allow that energy to come into the heart for self-love and passion.

Breathing is vitally important to humans. Breathing stands for life, and life stands for love and enjoyment. When people have breathing problems, asthma, or a weak heart, they are struggling to allow in their passion for life. Place the energy of amber exactly there—in the lungs, the bronchi, or the heart—to reignite the passion for life.

When allergies appear, always ask the question, "What am I really allergic to?" The magical amber energy, connected to the witches and guardians of the land, will help heal that vibration. Place amber wherever the allergy manifests physically and on the event or situations to which the person is allergic.

The ethereal crystal amber can easily be used to stimulate intuition and intelligence, clear the mind, and raise the vibration towards enlightenment.

# Amethyst

## *Purification*

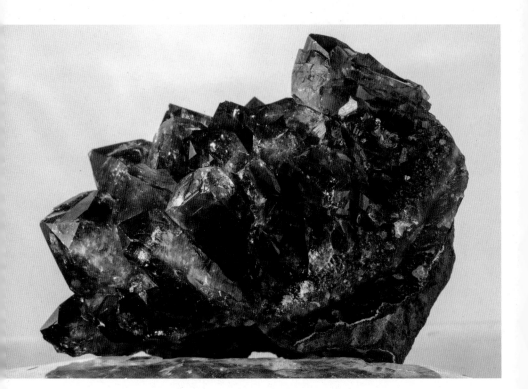

Amethyst energy purifies all energy. Amethyst energy is like an air purifier or a drop of washing-up liquid in a greasy pan. One puff and all vibrations clean up immediately. This ethereal crystal is very good to cleanse tense energies between people or in buildings.

To cleanse the energy between people after an argument, say, "Place amethyst between [name] and [name]."

To cleanse a room, say, "Place amethyst in this room." If you are not in that room, visualize the room, or just imagine the room by intention. Remember that there is no time or space. Creation is all in the intention.

The best known physical crystal amethyst comes in the colour purple. You can visualize the colour purple when using amethyst energy to purify, cleanse, relax, meditate, sleep, strengthen clairvoyance, or visualize better. Purple contains the colours red and blue—red is earth; blue is light. Thus, amethyst connects both aspects, Heaven and Earth, with each other. When we connect Heaven and Earth we rebalance, we realign.

Amethyst energy is relaxing, which is needed to make a connection with your higher self. This ethereal crystal brings bucket-loads of inner peace, inner harmony, and in its turn, clarity and insights.

If you work to purify matters of the heart or desire pure thoughts so you can create from the heart, you can visualize and tune into the vibration of green amethyst.

# Aquamarine

## *Wise Communication*

Aquamarine energy is there to help you step up! It is a wise, warm, and gentle vibration that works strongly on communication and creation. Aquamarine helps you find and express your feelings and intuition using the right words, an important step in the manifestation process. We need to be able to say what we want before we can receive it. Aquamarine can help with this.

Place aquamarine energy in the throat to heal the expression of thoughts and in the hands to create and receive magic. Aquamarine energy will help heal physical issues that manifest in the area between the nose and the thyroid. Say, "Place aquamarine in the thyroid", or "Place aquamarine in the sinuses."

Aquamarine can also be used to help improve hay fever symptoms. Place this energy in the throat and where the hay fever manifests physically. This vibration can also be placed between the person suffering from hay fever and Mother Earth.

If someone is afraid of being harmed by others, lacks trust, and does not feel safe, surround them with aquamarine vibrational energy to remind them that they are protected and always safe. Feeling unsafe is an illusion created by past experiences.

In its physical form, aquamarine ranges from light green to dark blue-green in colour, so this energy can easily be placed in the heart to connect with our higher purpose and take steps forward to create from the heart.

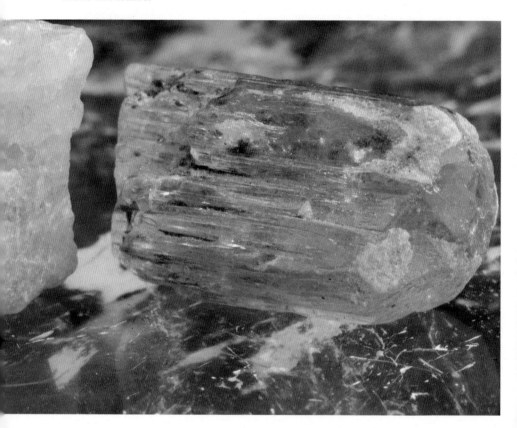

As aquamarine energy vibrates action, communication, and creation, you can place this energy between people when communication is hard or in the workspace to enhance trade, relationships, and business growth. Place this ethereal crystal around a person when they are in need of hope and their mood needs lifting. This ethereal crystal has high spiritual vibrations and can easily be used to channel a life purpose and attract the right business or work connections.

Place aquamarine energy around someone to strengthen their clairvoyant ability and allow them to open to higher spiritual vibrations consciously, especially during meditation.

# Aventurine

## *Choice*

The ethereal crystal aventurine is the energy to work with when decisions need to be made and emotions that are blocking the decision-making need to be healed. When we come to a crossroads, we need to know that whatever we choose is good for us. There is neither right nor wrong—only a decision and lessons that continue to guide us to where we need to be.

Trust that things will play out in divine perfection for you. If you notice that a certain decision isn't the right one, your soul still had to learn something. Once that has happened, it will be burnt into your consciousness and raise your vibration and that lower vibration will never be allowed into your creation again.

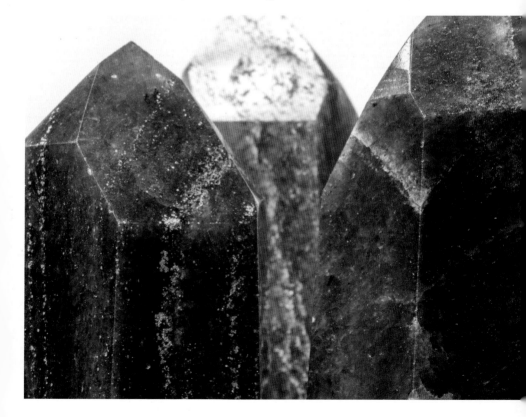

The ethereal crystal aventurine can be used as a shortcut to spiritual growth. Use its energy to help raise your vibration so you make the decision with the highest vibration and thus accelerate your spiritual growth. When aventurine helps you make decisions, it heals old karmic vibrations that may impede your decision-making. As you make "the best" decision, you step into the next level of vibration. As we are all connected, in doing so you instantly transform experiences and energy for everyone involved, in all directions of time and space.

Aventurine energy supports a woman in healing the deep wound of inequality between male and female by allowing them to experience a profound reconnection with femininity at the heart level. In this way, they heal the old pain of making decisions based on "not being enough" and not being seen for who they really are.

Using your intention, place this ethereal crystal in the hair follicles, the eyes, the heart, the hormones, and accept the female energy of receiving. Be patient, relaxed, courageous, tolerant, and optimistic about those who haven't woken up yet.

When working with aventurine, imagine the colour green. If you are drawn to it, you can also draw in red, orange, or light blue aventurine. Red is linked to the right to be female and powerful, orange to the need to make creative or sexual decisions, and light blue when needing to communicate with the ancestral line regarding female energy.

The vibration of aventurine works well for children and adults with a tendency towards aggression or simply for children who are busy and unsettled, as it allows their energy to go to their physical and mental growth instead of being wasted on anger.

On a physical level, aventurine can help heal skin issues, such as eczema, acne, other forms of skin rash, and red patches. Its healing vibration can also be placed in the hair follicles and scalp to help with dandruff and hair loss. Aventurine is a calming and pain-releasing ethereal crystal. Its vibration has a soothing effect on the physical heart, eyes, and fat metabolism.

Work with green aventurine when experiencing physical heart issues, such as palpitations and arrhythmias. It helps keep arteries open and thus prevents heart attacks.

# Calcite

*Growth*

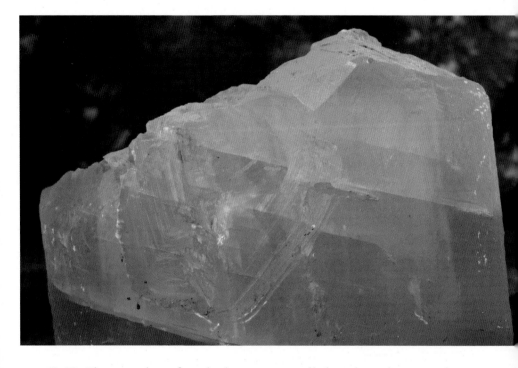

When you have found what you are called to do and want to be successful, work with the ethereal crystal calcite. You will most likely be drawn to the energy of calcite when you are ready to grow and build something lasting.

Working with calcite energy paves the path to success as it brings physical, mental, and spiritual growth. The path towards success and completion knows many different stages. Calcite will guide you and shine a light on what's important, when needed.

You can place the vibration of calcite in the workspace, the aura, the mind, the business, or in the physical body.

In the journey towards completion of any successful endeavour, you will encounter moments when you need motivation, self-confidence, hope, and courage. Trust the energy of calcite for help with healing old vibrations of wanting to give up, feelings of worthlessness, or the belief that something isn't for you. Stick with the energy of calcite to keep going and complete all in divine perfection for you.

The vibration of calcite brings together thoughts and feelings in a powerful and explosive way and serves as rocket fuel to accelerate the engine of growth and move things forward. The ability to move from initial desire to physical form necessarily involves growth. Calcite supports this on every level. Say, "Place calcite in the solar plexus" to receive vibrational healing and support.

Having an idea and the desire to see it accomplished is one thing, but if your energy is blocked and you lack the confidence, hope, and courage to move forward, it won't happen. Calcite will help heal that vibration. Yellow calcite, in particular, supports the strength of will necessary to get things done and the energy to do it.

Calcite not only assists the physical growth of children but also their mental and spiritual growth. Place calcite energy in the skeleton for optimal calcium intake, strength, and growth, and place this ethereal crystal in the elbows or brain to aid in concentration.

When your heart feels broken or hurt, place the energy of green calcite there for healing and growth, to raise the vibration, and let go of the old and move into a new level.

On a physical level, calcite energy helps heal the heart from rhythm defects, the heart in general, and stimulates the immune system.

# Chalcedony

*Trust and Flow*

An increasing number of humans have come to this planet to live several lives at once. These souls have decided to heal many things in just one lifetime, which should speed up the expansion of human consciousness. As a soul it looked easy enough, but once incarnated the soul forgot its life mission and now they are finding things incredibly hard. The vibration of chalcedony is here to support such people.

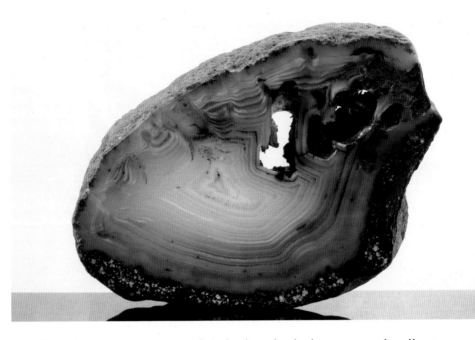

Working with the energy of chalcedony heals the emotions by allowing you to feel things deeply, face your emotions, let them go, and thus move to a new vibrational level. Chalcedony is a calm and gentle energy and perfect for children.

When my extremely premature daughter was born, chalcedony was the ethereal crystal I worked with most. She experienced a lot of oedema in her legs and female body parts. Oedema stands for holding on. She couldn't release the emotions she was feeling as she was afraid of letting go of her body, and the one thing she had to do to stay alive was keep her soul in her tiny body.

I placed chalcedony energy in the oedema in her legs and female parts with the strong intention to release that emotion in the perfect way. The vibration of chalcedony knows exactly how that needs to happen: trust. Chalcedony energy placed between a mother and child strengthens or heals the bond.

When you struggle to release emotions, you feel stuck in the past, reliving old emotions and creating the same old situations over and over. At that point there is no trust. The vibration of chalcedony helps you trust the flow of life and helps heal trauma, or rather, the emotions behind trauma. When you let go of the emotions, trauma no longer has a vibrational effect on you.

Depression, anger, and hopelessness are the result of emotions that were never dealt with. Say, "Place chalcedony in and around me, on every level of my being, in all directions of time and space."

We don't always need to know where our emotions and discomfort come from; we just need to change the vibration. Ethereal crystals represent "all that is"; as such, they know exactly where to go—in what strength, what colour, what form—to affect and heal the vibration—just like the wings of a butterfly, in all directions of time and space, everyone and everything involved.

Place the energy of the chalcedony in your aura to protect your pregnancy. And when struggling with tense relations between parents and children, say, "Place chalcedony between [name] and [name]."

As you release old emotions with the help of chalcedony, trust and flow can come in. Chalcedony energy helps you find your way.

Breathing also represents that flow, that joy. When there are issues with breathing and airways, say, "Place chalcedony on breathing and airways."

The ethereal crystal chalcedony supports emotional stability. Emotional stability creates higher vibration, trust, and flow, allowing new higher-vibrational things and experiences to flow into one's life.

# Chrysocolla
## *Calming*

The vibration of the ethereal crystal chrysocolla is here to soothe desperate humans. You ask, and you are given. You are the creator.

Life on Earth is an experience of opposites; there is a pro to every con. When people experience a con, they can get stuck in a downward spiral. Work with chrysocolla when things are peaking, as the vibration of this lovely ethereal crystal calms, balances, soothes, and helps create solutions.

Place the energy of chrysocolla between people when emotions are at a heart-breaking high; in the land and consciousness of war zones; in emotions and the heart when struggling to calm them; and in the feet when feeling angry with "life".

Chrysocolla ethereal crystal helps calm and reconnect us with our true self. When we experience peaks of emotion, anger, or physical pain, we have simply disconnected from our truth. Chrysocolla vibration will help change that. It literally is the answer to your cry for help.

On a physical level, chrysocolla helps heal arthritis, depression, rheumatism, backache, thyroid issues, PMS, hormonal issues, blood pressure, cramps, burn wounds, heart issues, lungs, metabolism, skin ulcers, tonsils, and throat infection.

All these physical issues have a sudden, strong peak of pain. Pain is experienced when we know in our soul how disconnected we are from our truth, but we have the need to punish ourselves out of embarrassment, guilt, or separation. Depending on where the physical pain is, it will

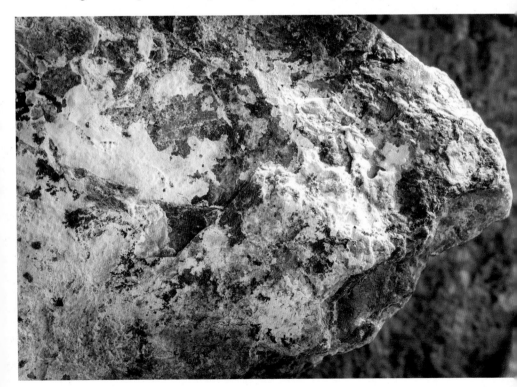

have another meaning. Arthritis, depression, rheumatism, and backache are linked to feeling separated from everything and everyone. Hormonal issues such as PMS, blood pressure, and cramps are linked to guilt and embarrassment. Heart, lung, and skin issues are a shout-out for love.

Another moment in life when we might experience a peak is when change presents itself. Even though change is the only constant in life, it is probably one of the hardest things for humans to deal with. We are creatures of habit—we like what we know.

When a change from the natural flow of things presents itself, it is an opportunity for evolution and expansion. Most humans, however, go against that and create a peak of guilt, shame, embarrassment, and separation. The energy of chrysocolla can be placed intentionally in the aura during meditation as a positive step forward in finding answers. It can also be placed in the aura, heart, or root chakra (energetically between the anus and genitalia) to encourage grounding, calm, and confidence.

# Citrine

## *Expansion*

Citrine vibration is present for those who are awakening. It is intricately linked with the energy of sunstone, and the two ethereal crystals work perfectly together. Citrine shows there is so much more out there than what you're currently experiencing. It helps break the metaphorical glass ceiling, so you can go beyond.

Citrine is here to remind you to go beyond what is, to expand. It is there to support you. If you feel there is a limit, tune into the energy of citrine, as it supports human consciousness to rise, allowing humanity to leave the old limited vibrational plane behind and ascend to the next one, embracing life beyond physical boundaries. Citrine says, "Who is with me? Let's go!"

The vibration of citrine offers a major energy boost. When you are feeling tired or listless, place the energy of the citrine in your solar plexus by saying, "Place citrine in the solar plexus", pointing at your stomach.

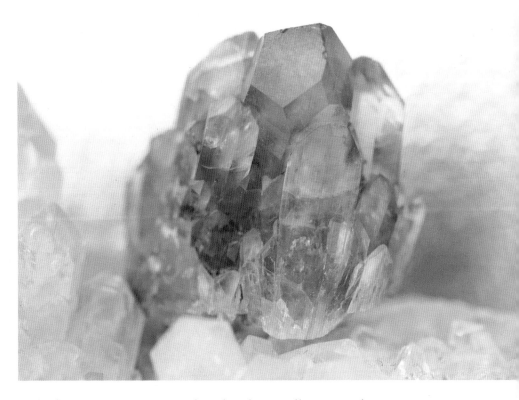

Placing citrine energy in the solar plexus will improve the energy stream in all organs. Depending on where expansion is needed, you can call in different-coloured citrine ethereal crystals. For example, use green citrine for expansion of the heart, love, and self-love.

Citrine vibration can create fabulous results on a blocked sacral chakra and solar plexus, which are linked to trouble with the right to feel and the right to act. Place citrine in the belly and on the stomach to address these issues.

Citrine energy symbolizes the sun and the light in all of us. It is the ideal ethereal crystal to work with when in need of mental and energetic support. Say, "Place citrine in [name/my] mind", or "Place citrine around [name/me]."

Citrine will give a sudden burst of energy and improve the energy stream in all organs. This vibration strengthens endurance and has a positive influence on the nervous system.

Citrine connects you with your own power.

# Clear Quartz

*Unity*

Clear quartz ethereal crystal contains the vibration of pilgrims, seekers, and enlightened souls. It is available to bring more light into Earth's consciousness and human minds.

Clear quartz energy is the purest energy of all. White contains all colours. It sheds light on and can heal any situation. Clear quartz has an incredible healing capacity and gives off pure light energy. This vibration is available so we can raise our energy and just be, then send that vibration of light out so it affects other people and encourages them to do the same thing; lift vibration, shine, and energetically affect others to do the same. The more light we create, the better for everyone.

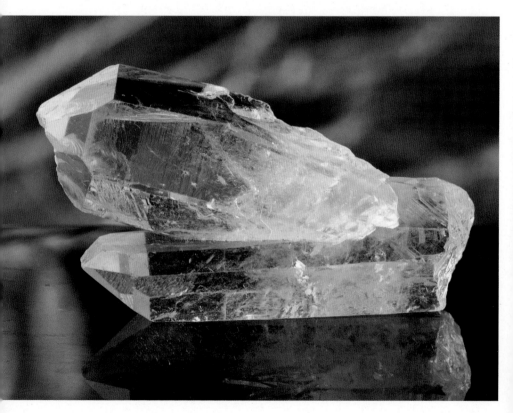

At first, you may struggle to work with the energy of clear quartz as it is so bright. If that's the case, it's better to use it in combination with a grounding ethereal crystal. One of the signs that you are not ready to use clear quartz alone is a feeling of light-headedness, as if you are on another planet. If you experience this, use smoky quartz instead or clear quartz in combination with a grounding ethereal crystal, such as jasper, onyx, agate, or ruby.

This can be compared with turning the light on in a pitch-black room or sunlight coming in through the crack between the curtains. This is what the vibration of clear quartz does—it helps overcome fear and brings light to the mind and body of anyone struggling with depression. It stimulates clear thinking and literally "turns on the light"; it stimulates physical and mental stability.

Say, "Place clear quartz in the solar plexus", or "Place clear quartz in the root chakra" to remove the darkness someone experiences. You can also say, "Place clear quartz in [room]" to cleanse a heavy atmosphere.

Physically, the energy of clear quartz helps heal backache, bleeding, diarrhoea, and the physical heart.

Place the vibration of clear quartz in the solar plexus and root chakra when suffering from car and sea sickness. It will help ground and equalize the energy throughout the body.

Menopause or menstruation problems indicate a struggle with cycles, change, and flow. By working with the vibration of clear quartz, you clear the path. It is as if you are on a dusty, bumpy road full of old leaves and branches that came down during a storm. The storm represents emotional pain that made you not trust the path and flow anymore. By placing the energy of clear quartz, we turn the light on in a pitch-black room. Clear quartz cleans up the old emotional hang-ups with the snap of the fingers.

After an illness, or as a spring cure, use your intention to place a clear quartz Triangle shape with the point downwards with the spoken intention to keep the crystal energy there for up to two weeks to help cleanse the body. To boost mental energy and prevent tiredness, use your intention to place the clear quartz Triangle with the point upwards. When the point is downwards it is for cleansing; when it is upwards it radiates energy to the mind and body.

# Emerald

*Passion*

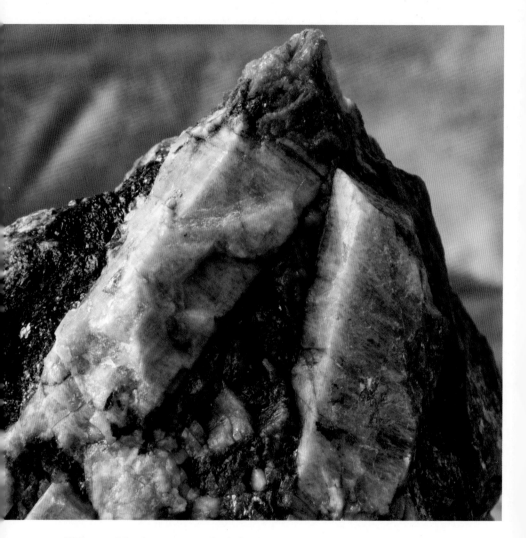

Emerald vibration is ideal for lonely, romantic souls as a means to create love, romance, connection, and unity. This ethereal crystal reminds us that love comes from within our own hearts, and to experience love, we need to reconnect with the love in our own hearts first. It brings the cocktail of all we need to find that love again:

- Healing tears by acknowledging them
- Seeing the illusion and understanding that it was all just an experience
- Taking responsibility and healing the heart will make it overflow with love.

Emerald is the symbol of true love, inspiration, and positivity. When the heart is healing, everything else in life can heal and physical experiences can transform. The outside world and personal experience are merely a reflection of the inside world.

Working with the energy of emerald supports spiritual healing. When the heart aches because it has been forced to love the Church more than our own hearts; when we were forced to love a man or woman who was not meant for us; when we were forced to see things that were the opposite of love—emerald helps it heal. Emerald heals melancholy, the emotion created by humans after experiencing deep pain on a heart level. I am sure it is obvious as well that the vibration of emerald creates passion.

Physically, emerald energy helps with recuperation after an illness and helps heal the eyes, rheumatism, epilepsy, the heart, and the immune system. For the strengthening of the immune system, say, "Place emerald on the coccyx, heart, and above the head."

After suffering at the hands of spiritual or religious institutions or followers of spiritual or religious institutions, tune into emerald to help heal. Say, "Place emerald above my head."

You can also draw emerald vibration into Mother Earth where the events took place or place the vibration on the event. The event does not need to be visualized; it is all about intention, and directing emerald vibration to where it is needed is enough.

When experiencing claustrophobia or depression, the passionate energy of emerald can really support in uplifting vibration and creating new passion within. Emerald is a gorgeous energy to meditate with and helps activate clairvoyance.

# Fluorite

## *Ascension*

Fluorite is to be found in all the colours of the rainbow. If you work with intention, the Universe will give you the best colour, as the Universe is all-knowing.

Several times, when I was offering chakra healing, my gut told me to place fluorite on the root chakra, which is all about grounding, trust, and confidence.

At first, I found this quite confusing as fluorite energy is so high-vibration, but it makes sense now. Fluorite vibration lines you up with Heaven and Earth, male and female, past and present, giving and receiving. Fluorite will always help you in whatever growth stage you are in. Fluorite works on the auric layers and consciousness.

Many children nowadays experience difficult parental behaviour and may also have trouble with concentration and learning problems. Meanwhile, many more adults have life-threatening illnesses like cancer. Those issues most often have their roots in past-life experiences, when people were told the opposite of what they were experiencing and children were not allowed to ask questions or think for themselves.

Throughout previous lives, people have experienced war, violence, and other horrific things, and this past energy stays within the psyche and energy system. It is because of this that many children these days have concentration problems, bad memories, nightmares, and may also suffer from depression.

Fluorite is an ethereal crystal that offers beautiful healing and supports the release of energies we can't consciously remember. It balances the left and right hemispheres of the brain and enables clarity of thought and concentration. It is perfect for people, especially children, who have had paranormal experiences that have left them feeling unsettled and nervous. Fluorite helps tone down the impressions left by these experiences and fosters acceptance. The energy of this ethereal crystal calms those who use a lot of energy physically and mentally and is particularly useful for those who are consciously working on their inner growth process.

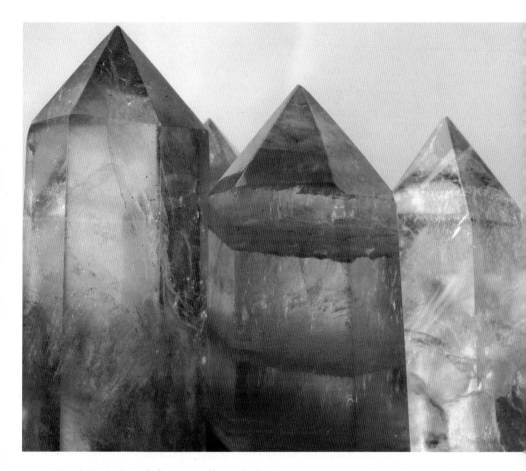

The vibration of fluorite allows balance to be restored. It boosts the ability to speak with confidence in a group and harmonizes feelings and thoughts to create emotional balance.

Physically, fluorite is a supportive energy to bring in when undergoing a major operation; it works positively on bone marrow, cells, and diseases such as leukaemia or any other cancer. It can also help improve outcomes when it comes to donating blood. After giving blood, say, "Place fluorite in this blood", and point at the bag containing your blood. Imagine the person who needs a blood transfusion receiving your blood, now strengthened with the hugely powerful vibration of fluorite. What a gift of life that is!

Fluorite also positively supports the healing of communication through the throat, nose, ears, brain tissues, and mental functions.

# Garnet

## *Treasure*

The vibration of garnet helps widows heal their broken hearts, open to feeling passion again, and allow themselves to once more feel the warmth, body, and love of a man or woman after losing their partner. In the past, many strong wives had to hold their families together, work the land, and feed the children after their husbands died. The strength and willpower of garnet are beyond measure. It is pure fire and power.

The inventiveness and strength of garnet energy in times of need can also be used to locate your treasure; the deepest of passions within can be found and extracted by working with garnet. When you don't know your calling or your soul's purpose, surround yourself with the energy of garnet ethereal crystal.

Do not use garnet if you have high blood pressure! Because of its incredible strength it could make blood pressure rise even more. If you have low blood pressure, though, this crystal can be helpful.

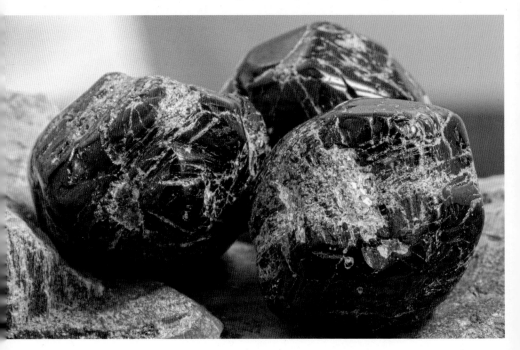

Garnet is an ethereal crystal associated with the grounding energy of the heart. By this, I mean that it taps heart energy and brings what's in the heart into consciousness. In this way, pain can be given space and released, strength can be found, and treasure can come to light.

On a physical level, garnet crystal helps heal heart issues, strengthens the heart, and helps rebalance the heart's rhythm. Ethereal crystal garnet helps regulate the heartbeat physically and emotionally and helps heal skin conditions.

People suffering from depression have pretended to be someone they're not for way too long—who they are has been "depressed", or pushed down. Garnet can guide them on the journey to finding their treasure and life purpose, grounding it in their consciousness, and finding the strength, confidence, and rootedness to rise to their purpose.

As garnet carries so much strength, it also carries a lot of passion. This energy can help light the flame of passion within relationships. Say, "Place garnet between [name] and [name]." Place it on the heart level or pelvic level.

The emotions that underlie anger and angry outbursts are sadness, loneliness, and pain. By surrounding the body with garnet, we can reconnect with the warm self, heal sadness and loneliness, and release anger.

Garnet energy encourages, energizes, and as it supports you in finding your soul's purpose, helps you walk the path towards success.

# Hematite

### *Energetic Buffer*

Hematite is the divinely perfect vibration for nurses and carers. Hematite builds a see-through wall around a person, so they are seen but all lower and negative vibrations from others bounce off the wall and back to the sender. In this way, the person enveloped by hematite is protected.

This ethereal crystal is perfect for those who must do a lot of listening to the problems and whining of other people. It makes them strong and patient without being affected by what they hear.

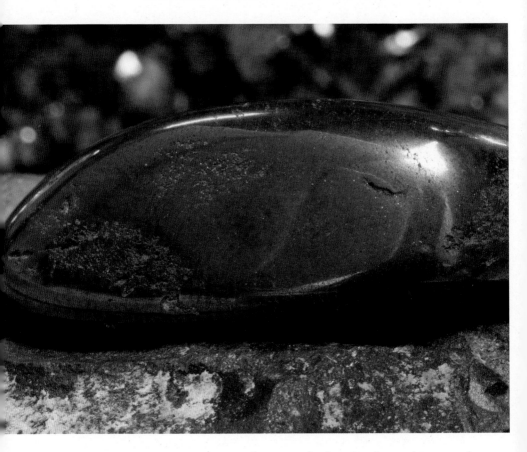

Hematite supports us during the proverbial storm by making us the eye of the storm, with the ability to stay calm, collected, and grounded during crazy times. Hematite is a grounding energy and gives deep roots. These are needed if we want to stand strongly when navigating challenging times.

When you are having difficulty sleeping due to restlessness brought on by stress, hematite will calm you and bring you back into your body and allow peaceful sleep.

Hematite is a support for anyone experiencing physical weakness as it strengthens body and mind. Hematite energy is a natural homeostatic, which makes it an ideal healer of the blood. It's an enormously powerful vibration for people suffering from life-threatening illnesses. To work with it, say, "Place hematite in the blood." Even for simple things like wounds, place hematite energy there for quick healing.

# Jasper

*Anchor*

Jasper energy is present for the fearful, those souls that want to escape being human and struggle to just be and enjoy life. Jasper is here for those who fear the mind and let that run their lives, instead of anchoring themselves mentally and working with trust to take positive control.

Jasper is an ethereal crystal that offers real connection with Mother Earth. It places the feet of people and animals firmly on the ground, makes fear go away, and creates space for security and confidence. As a result, we can find ourselves again, appreciate ourselves, and open to other people.

Many people have taken on human lives hundreds, even thousands, of times in the past, but the consciousness and vibrations back then were too low to allow most to wake up, so they experienced pain, physical limitations, and emotional, physical, and spiritual violence and they

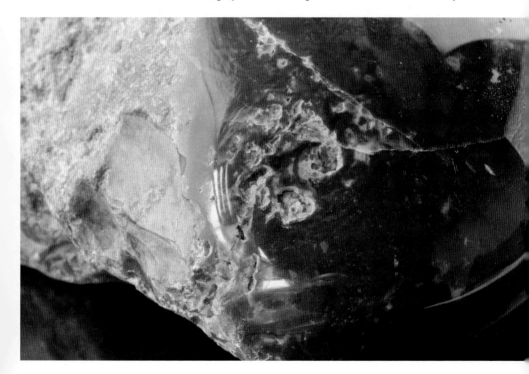

disconnected from life. In other words, they cut off their roots, and when a tree has no roots, it dies and falls to the ground.

In order to feel confident, strong-willed, and receive the nutrients of life—support, guidance, happiness, money, and love—humans need roots, for the feet to be anchored to Mother Earth. Jasper offers exactly that—to be.

Say, "Place jasper in the feet", then "see" roots come out of your feet and nestle deeply into the planet. The roots can then glow with the reddish-brown colour of jasper. They can also be imagined as yellow to feel confident to act upon your life purpose or green to deeply love life.

This ethereal crystal is an incredible support for people suffering from pregnancy sickness. Say, "Place jasper in the stomach", or "Place jasper on the endocrine system."

Jasper can help bring back your sense of smell if it has been lost. Using the ethereal crystal, you literally say, "Place jasper on my sense of smell", then trust that the vibration is placed where needed to heal any sense of smell issues.

Jasper aids with the bladder, in general, as well as bladder infections. Say, "Place jasper in the bladder."

Jasper also works well for liver issues. The liver helps detoxify drugs and alcohol; produces bile needed for digestion; stores micronutrients; and helps the immune system, blood clotting, and cholesterol transport. In other words, the liver has a huge function.

Now let me translate this:

- Anger is the emotion linked to a malfunctioning liver.
- Drugs and alcohol are a desperate way to numb emotions.
- The liver produces bile for good digestion. Anger comes up when we're not digesting situations properly, when we don't know how to.
- Micronutrients are needed to nourish, to feed the body, to make it thrive. When we're angry, all self-nutrition flies out of the window.
- Anger diminishes the immune system as we damage it through high stress levels.
- Blood clotting issues are linked to anger and running away from undigested situations.

Jasper can be worked with for all the above-mentioned issues. It allows you to anchor yourself, digest emotions, allow the nutrients of life into the body and life experience, feel confident and protected in every situation, and ground deeply in the body and life.

Physically, jasper ethereal crystal also protects against strokes and epilepsy. Say, "Place jasper in the third eye" and "Place jasper in the head." To anchor yourself in place instead of escaping, say, "Place jasper in the feet." You can choose a specific colour of jasper to add even more power. If you're not sure, don't worry—the Universe will automatically choose the right colour.

# Labradorite

## *Salvation*

The vibration of labradorite is one of pure higher-power energy. It is connected with Indigo and Crystal children and knocking down institutions and programmes and building new ones.

Indigo children are headstrong and will need this "I am not giving in" attitude throughout their lives, as they have come to Earth to smash the old way of doing things. They often have difficult childhoods and are old souls that know exactly how life on Earth works. Most are now adults. Crystal children started coming to Earth slightly after the Indigos. Their energy is light, and most of them haven't been human before, or only once or twice. Their energy is pure, honest, and one of pure love. These souls came to rebuild Earth after the Indigos smashed the old.

Indigos remove the old foundation; Crystals build a new one. As such, labradorite is a beautiful energy with which to surround an Indigo or Crystal child so that they feel supported on their journey.

Labradorite ethereal crystal can be placed around anything in need of transformation. In this way, outdated patterns will show themselves and be removed or changed, making way for the creation of something new and a thousand times better.

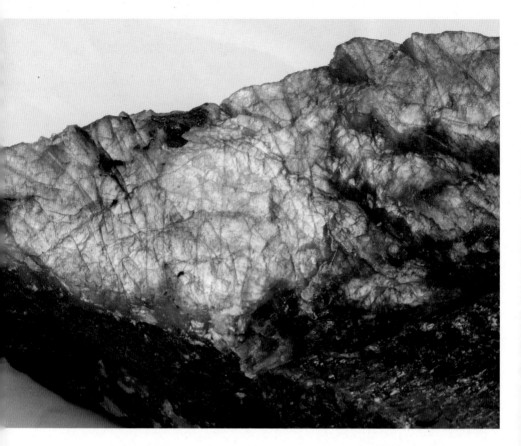

Work with labradorite when a business is struggling or looking to explore new and improved avenues. Say, "Place labradorite on the spine of [name of the business]", "Place labradorite in the centre of [name of the business]", or "Place labradorite around [name of the business]." Use labradorite on the spine when a business needs to undergo a transformation, such as changing the makeup of its trustees, board, and financiers or when the founder has died and the business is trying to find the best way forward. Use the same technique to help transform homes and relationships.

Labradorite is of huge value for the healing of the aura as it is an exceptional protector. If someone has been battling disease or heavy emotional or psychological problems, labradorite will heal the weak places in the aura with strong, beautiful energy so the body is restored and full of light, strength, and love.

# Lapis Lazuli

*Friendship*

Lapis lazuli is a beautiful, gentle vibration with which to create. The physical crystal exists in diverse tints of blue, most of the time with gold-coloured specks. It stands for golden communication. When communicating openly with the self, the deepest truths can be communicated with the Universe and the Universe can bring you what you asked for. People underestimate the importance of communication with the self. We cannot receive our desires in physical form if we don't communicate them properly with the Universe, and we cannot communicate our true desire with the Universe if we don't communicate with our deepest self first.

To communicate with our deepest self, we must first calm, ground, and connect with our body. Lapis lazuli placed in the feet, mind, and/ or around us can really help with this, as this crystal represents calm, balance, and communication.

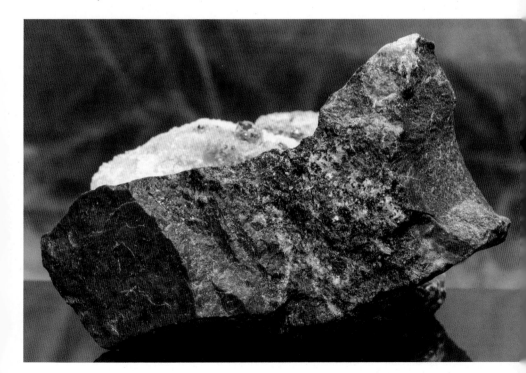

Lapis lazuli is the friendship crystal and is ideal for attracting new friendships and easy-flowing, divinely perfect connections.

When there is no inspiration or energy left to take steps forward due to embarrassment or fear of being seen, we can feel left exhausted, lacking strength and will, unable to sleep, and low in mental energy. Place the energy of lapis lazuli around the bed to help with getting to sleep and recovery while asleep. Place lapis lazuli in the solar plexus in order to send equal energy around the body, to the meridians, organs, blood vessels, and brain, to feel energized physically and mentally.

Lapis lazuli supports anything and everything that needs "growing", such as money, friendships, confidence, energy, intuition, happiness, and being seen. Invite lapis lazuli in and around you if you want to transform your life.

Physically, lapis lazuli also protects against stroke.

Allergies, problems with nerves, and depression have their roots in not trusting life, feeling cut off and alone, and feeling inner anger for it. Lapis lazuli can make a real difference when it comes to these diseases. This ethereal crystal can help find trust, connection, and calm again. As a result, healing from depression, nerve issues, and allergies can take place and new seeds of desires can be sown, nurtured, and grow.

When we experience fear and uncertainty, it can make us feel angry. When we are unable to find ourselves or friends or love ourselves, it can bring problems with the nervous and immune systems in the body. Lapis lazuli is the right ethereal crystal to work with!

# Malachite

## *Empress*

Malachite brings young, unfolding, and controlled energy, but its core explodes with true magic, seduction, warmth, respect, wildness, and mesmerizing vibrations. Malachite stands for new beginnings and creation, such as a new baby, job, or relationship. The main message of malachite is that it brings physical enjoyment. It is a versatile ethereal crystal.

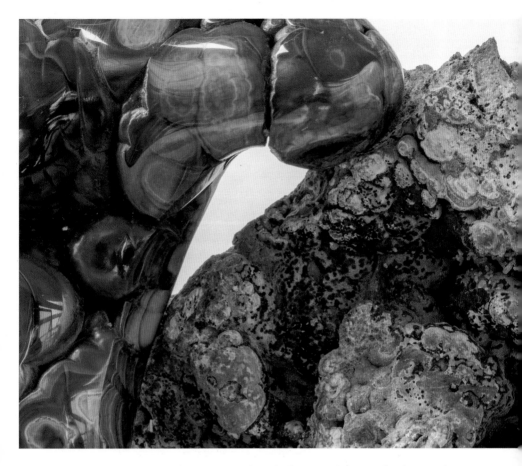

Malachite cleanses and balances the chakras and reminds those who are fully conscious, of the meaning of Source: love and enjoyment. It is for those who want to remember and live life the way it is intended by Source—with flow, trust, and physical enjoyment.

Malachite is an ethereal crystal that allows women to rediscover their sexuality, pleasure, and receptivity. Whether it be the loss of zest for life, creative will or will to physically create babies, enjoyment of the physical delights that sexual contact brings, or the power of orgasms and youthful pleasure at every stage of life, malachite heals and guides. Placing malachite vibration in the womb (for women) or prostate (for men) will help reignite that vibration.

When we give ourselves permission to feel, receive, and create, we connect with the essence of life, and true magic can enter life.

So many women have gone into survival mode. To be honest, throughout history, they have had to become independent and sort things out for themselves. Men would die young and women would have to bring up huge families, or men would be so traumatized by war and violence they could no longer give anything. So women had to be the backbone of the family and society, all the while carrying the trauma of not being protected in their wombs.

As you now know, a woman is a receiver and must be given to, but how can they be open and receive if they are not protected? A woman can be independent and strong but must also be allowed to show vulnerability. Vulnerability is a strength not a weakness, but it can only be felt and shown when they feel safe. Healed men can handle vulnerability. Healed men give, don't take. Healed men will always do everything they can to support their women, give to them, and be there for them in their vulnerability.

Men can work with this energy, too. Both men and women have been affected by life, resulting in a huge imbalance between male and female, giving and receiving, thus both can work with malachite to restore that balance.

Tune into malachite to restore money flow, a male energy that pertains to giving. As they take on male energy, strong, independent women have started giving and stopped receiving, and as a result, suddenly find themselves having impeded financial flow. Restoring the true female energy of "receiving" can help restore money flow energy.

Bone issues are linked to a "wobbly structure" in your being. So many women struggle with osteoarthritis, arthritis, fractures, and brittle bones once they start menopause. This is because they had to give so much to their families, work, and life that suddenly, as they transition, their structure falls apart. But women aren't givers, they are receivers! If women would stay in their natural receiving mode, that wouldn't happen. Malachite can help with prevention at a younger age and support healing after women turn 40. Malachite energy can be channelled into the aura, the mind, the womb, the prostate, the heart (to receive), and the bones.

Physically, malachite ethereal crystal helps heal fractures and liver problems, reduces cramps and high blood pressure, and supports the processing of trauma. For this last one, place malachite in the mind, and/or on the connection between the person and the traumatic event and/or persons involved.

Place malachite ethereal crystal in former war zones to reestablish balance and heal men and women, so that men can give from the heart again and women are safe to receive.

As the ethereal crystal malachite is a female energy, it is a huge support for menstruation problems, female sex hormones, childbirth, and getting to the root of sexual problems with psychological roots.

When balance is disturbed, it literally makes us "spin". The body reacts to the mind, and once the dominant vibration becomes strong enough, the body always manifests it physically. When the vibration is out of balance, in "fight or flight" mode, the physical results can be dizziness, epilepsy, car sickness, and restrictive behavioural and thinking patterns as a desperate attempt to find balance. Malachite will help restore balance.

As explained earlier, that imbalance came about because women had to be strong and independent as the result of trauma. Malachite can help process trauma, whether that's in the conscious mind or in past lives.

# Moonstone

## Creation

Moonstone is the female ethereal crystal that will bring men in contact with their emotional side. This ethereal crystal belongs to love, gods, goddesses, and propagation.

Women have been whisked away from their cycle and taught to jump on the crazy merry-go-round of life. Men and women were both taught to work until they drop every day and that rest is for the weak and the dead.

Moonstone vibration is here to remind us to walk the land, to connect with the planet through our bare feet. It is here to remind us of the seasons, to plant the seed and wait patiently, trusting that the flower will bloom or the wheat grow. It is here to remind us that the earth prepares, nurtures and grows, blooms, dies, and rests.

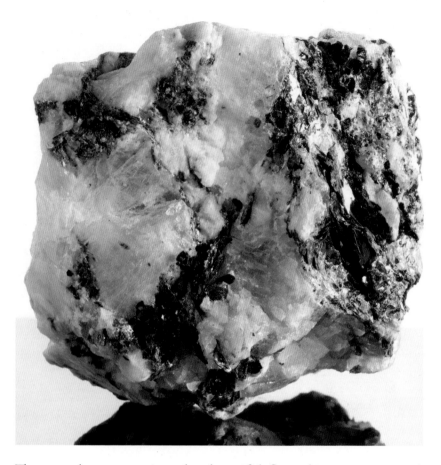

The second we go against that beautiful flow, things go wrong. A perfectly gorgeous apple will not taste sweet and juicy when impatience makes us pick the apple before it's ripe. Human eyes will never see the lush colours of the flowers if they continually mow them down and as a result, bees and birds never find them, go hungry, and die. One small action of not trusting the cycle can disturb the whole cycle. Nature and the Universe will continue to find a way to bring about results and restart new cycles, and that is also something moonstone ethereal crystal brings—the restarting of the perfect cycles for you, time and time again. Every day brings new chances.

Women struggle to conceive because they have disconnected from "receiving mode". Women struggle with menstruation problems because they forget, or have never been taught, to rest. Women have hormonal problems because they are afraid to let go. The cycle has been disturbed and pushed aside. Absolutely everything in life has a cycle. Here are the different stages:

*Preparation – Conception – Spring – Maiden – First Quarter Moon*

*Bloom – Expression – Summer – Woman – New Moon*

*Releasing – Letting Go – Autumn – Last Quarter Moon – Wise Woman*

*Winter – Rest – Contemplation – Death – Transformation – Full Moon*

Moonstone can help us to reconnect with the cycle that is a part of all life.

As noted, this ethereal crystal is not only for women. Men are also inhabitants of this planet and part of its cycles, so they too must prepare, bloom, let go, and rest. This is the one constant in life: cycles.

Let's compare it with water. Water will start gorgeously fresh at its spring headwaters, then debouche into a fast, flowing river. It will let go as it crashes down a waterfall and eventually flow calmly through the woods.

Or take the sun. The sun appears in the morning sky in a flood of gorgeous, glowing colours and cool temperatures. As it rises, so does the temperature, and it glows and shines brightly through the day. In late afternoon, it starts to fade and let go of its strength. Eventually, at sunset, it "disappears" and "rests" until it comes back the next day and the cycle starts all over again.

Cycles are a part of creation. Without them, there is no creation. Humans can't bloom without preparation, letting go, and rest. Moonstone helps us remember to reconnect with the cycles, thus this energy helps us to create again, whether it be sexuality, projects, babies, emotions, happiness, success, or abundance.

Water retention, constipation, emotional issues, mood swings, PMS, cellulite, stress, fear, intoxication, stomach problems, and digestive issues are all signs of not being able to let go. Without letting go, there can be no rest; without rest, we can't create anything new. Moonstone can help heal those physical issues. It is also a brilliant guide for healing muscle weakness and obesity.

# Morganite

*Movement*

Morganite is for those striving to bring about change. This ethereal crystal supports the slightly frustrated humans who see the stagnation of humanity and see the comfort zones people get stuck in. Morganite helps shift and move stuff, especially matters of the heart.

Unpleasant experiences from earlier lives can affect the heart without people even realizing. Blockages here can be carried into our next lives, leading to serious physical, emotional, and psychological problems. By calling on morganite, we can erase these blockages, let go of past vibrations, and create beautiful, free, loving, healthy heart experiences—love and be loved.

Morganite heals in a gentle way, deeply and instantly. It helps heal every layer so you can let go and transform into a positive person and live in the here and now.

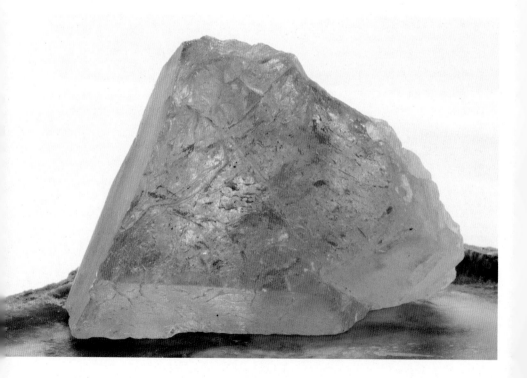

Humans easily get stuck in old stories—what happened during child-hood, what their father or mother did, the neighbour who didn't like them, the girlfriend who couldn't commit. People relive that emotional vibration day after day and become that emotion.

Have you ever heard someone say their friend is a sad person. No one is sad; this person just went through a life experience that was very sad, never dealt with the emotions fully, and relives the emotion day after day and now has become the emotion: sadness, living in sadness every day, "being a sad person". In other words, the emotion of sadness got stuck. The emotion of sadness didn't shift and move out and has now become this person's predominant vibration.

Morganite brings strength, hope, change, and growth. This is an especially important ethereal crystal for these times. We need to move things forward, out of the old into the new.

Physically, morganite ethereal crystal heals stomach issues, digestive problems, muscular problems, heart issues, and anything to do with the legs.

# Obsidian

## *Now*

Obsidian shows us the truth of how and what things really are. This ethereal crystal works like a magnet, transforming the powers of the mind into clear, active power.

Obsidian is indeed extremely powerful, and it is only to be used in a positive way: to turn visions into reality and trust that what materializes is for your highest good.

A very long time ago, the physical crystal obsidian was used in black magic to manipulate and force others to do things. We can learn a great deal from obsidian vibration, but it can only be worked with by those who know and respect this ethereal crystal's extraordinary powers.

Harness obsidian energy for meditation, manifestation, grounding, and living in the here and now. This ethereal crystal enables the power

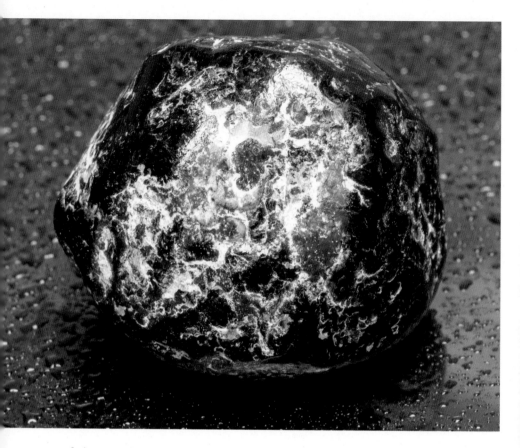

of the mind to be grounded, opening doors to personal possibilities. At the same time, it allows all illusion to disappear so only the truth survives.

It is only in darkness that seeds grow, and obsidian brings that vibration and manifestation. Often, when people feel as though they want to die, they don't realize they don't want to do so physically; it is their spirit that is ready for transformation! The old wants to die so that the new can come in. When you feel you're in a dark time, work with obsidian. You would not feel this pain unless you were really ready to transform. This also means that the seeds for something new are also there, sitting in that darkness, ready to open and grow.

After meditating with obsidian, make sure to always bring back the balance by placing a Clear Crystal shape around you to perfectly balance darkness and light.

When you are releasing curses or past life contracts, place obsidian on the contracts and mind of all involved in all directions of time and space for immediate effect.

As with onyx, I wouldn't use a physical black crystal for children, as it is too heavy to bear, but I have noticed that you can safely use black ethereal crystals on children. That's because the Universe always gives off just the right vibration for each person; it will know the obsidian is for a child, and thus choose a light obsidian holding the divinely perfect vibration.

You can also choose to use rainbow obsidian. This obsidian offers all of the obsidian qualities for healing as well as the positivity, hope, and happiness of rainbow light contained in that ethereal crystal.

# Onyx

## *Liberation*

Deep, warm, comforting, and sometimes painful yet liberating onyx vibration is the perfect ethereal crystal for mourning. Onyx energy supports widows, mothers who have lost children, and all who mourn and need to release their grief.

This ethereal crystal contains all of the colours and stages of grief, allowing you to move through each one deeply and swiftly while staying grounded and connected with the earth. In this way, Mother Earth—life—can help heal and transmute the energy that is released and raise the vibration.

When we are liberated from grief, our hearts can open and our intuition be heard again, so that we can see the beauty of life and hear the tender voices of our loved ones.

The physical onyx crystal is black with thin layers of white. Sometimes it has thin brown sides. Those are the colours you can visualize when you tune into this energy.

This is an immensely powerful ethereal crystal as it travels to the deepest crevices of the heart. No matter what emotional pain formed our grief, it must be released so that it cannot fester. Using onyx for healing gives the grief space so it can be felt and supported. We live in a world of opposites; feeling grief shows how much love there is. Onyx vibration also helps restore good energy flow when grief has paralyzed us. Onyx offers an incredible connection with Mother Earth!

Tap into ethereal crystal onyx in order to help with matters of the heart—the physical heart, the emotional heart, and the heart's intuition.

Specific physical issues onyx can help heal include problems with the airways, asthma, lungs, teary eyes, and deafness. Onyx also helps heal skin problems. The skin stands for feeling the outside world. When skin problems appear, it means that grief and emotional pain must be released. Say, "Place onyx on [skin issues], and place onyx on [emotions]." Trust the process.

When the heart is blocked due to emotional pain and grief, our hearing will also shut down. By "hearing", I mean both the physical ears and the intuition, the inner ear. By working with the energy of onyx

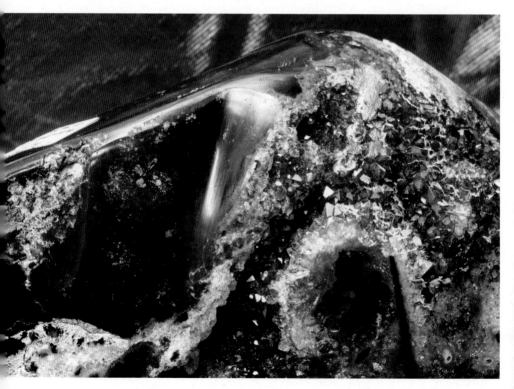

ethereal crystal, you can release the roots of the emotional pain and grieving and, in this way, allow yourself to listen to and hear your own voice and those of others so that you can reconnect with the self and the loving world around you.

People who are grieving frequently struggle with daily tasks. By healing the grief and painful emotions (read: processing them and giving them a place), you improve concentration, live increasingly in the here-and-now, and allow enjoyment to enter again.

When someone struggles to love and be loved and is afraid and uncertain about love and being loved, onyx is a magical ethereal crystal to work with.

Note: When children are grieving, it often is better to choose rose quartz (see below). Trust your intuition.

# Rose Quartz

## *Gentleness*

Rose quartz is a beautiful, gentle, loving energy to work with. It tells you that you have the right to love and be loved. You can imagine it in your mind's eye as the colour pink.

Ethereal crystal rose quartz is a perfect energy to place in the bedroom of children of all ages, from babies to teenagers. Its vibration is ideal for babies, as it helps them gently adjust to life on Earth at their own pace. I would place the energy of rose quartz around the baby's crib or in the baby's aura.

The gentle pink energy of rose quartz helps children of all ages stay true to each life stage and not grow up too fast; it keeps a childlike atmosphere. Its pink colour is protective and heals the energy of the heart.

In adults, this energy heals a broken heart that has left us shut down, hardened, not believing that "all is for the best, and being tough is the way to be". Rose quartz energy will allow the heart to open to the beauty of life once again. Imagine that energy in your heart; really pull it in. It will help you rediscover that gentle feeling within yourself. If you are an

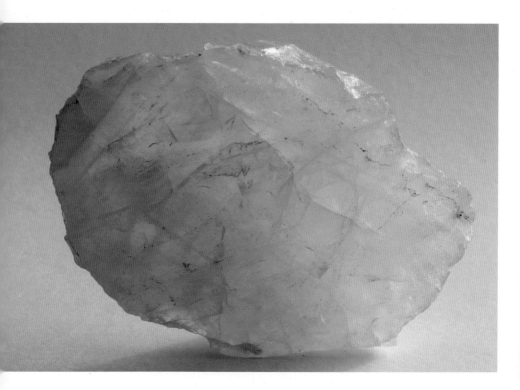

adult who has built a wall around you, or don't know how to be playful anymore, working with the energy of rose quartz will help you soften, smile, relax, and find that innocent child energy again.

Note: When you feel that you need rose quartz energy but know that the wall you've built around yourself or the gentle energy you've pushed away was caused by pain, rose quartz can cause emotional outbursts while healing takes place. This is because working with rose quartz energy allows those rejected feelings and forgotten memories to resurface for healing. When they pop up, it's because they are ready, and you are ready, for them to be released.

Allow those old emotions to resurface and feel them. Try to feel them as if they are just visiting, and they're on their way out. Feel them, see them, maybe even thank them for the lessons, and say goodbye to them. This is part of the healing process instigated and guided by rose quartz energy. Trust the powerful gentleness of rose quartz.

Once the old is released and you continue to work with the energy of rose quartz, you can form a different relationship with this energy.

Your relationship with yourself and things in your emotional world will truly transform.

Rose quartz teaches us to love ourselves, and loving ourselves is crucial. If we are dreaming of a divine love relationship, we must start with the love we feel for ourselves, with unconditional love for the self, or self-love with no conditions attached! Once we can do that, we can open up to a partner who also loves themselves unconditionally and has a healthy relationship with themselves (or they are deeply working on that). Then you will attract a truly perfect love relationship. Rose quartz energy can help with self-love and attracting the perfect partner. Place it by intention in your heart, your mind, and all around you.

You can also use your intention to place rose quartz energy in your legs and consciously walk lovingly, restoring your bond with earthly life. Many people don't trust life. Past lives or this current life have only brought pain, such as lack of money and safety. This is all within the "earthly bond". To be given all earthly needs, you need a strong bond with earthly life. This is also love. Rose quartz can help restore that energy, that bond.

Rose quartz energy is inspiring for creative people. It can be placed in the mind to stimulate the imagination and in the heart or throat to stimulate expression. Use your intention to place rose quartz energy around your workstation or fill your workspace with this gorgeous light energy.

Rose quartz can have a magical healing effect on the physical body. To place this energy in your nervous system, just say, "Place rose quartz in my nervous system." Or you can pull the ethereal crystal into your body by looking at the image of rose quartz, seeing and feeling its vibrant pink energy. Trust that! You don't need to know detailed anatomy in order to heal. It's all in your intention. The wisdom of ethereal crystals in combination with your positive intention knows what to do.

Physical uses include for blood circulation, breasts, heart, blood, lungs, arms, hands, upper back, and the release of impurities from body fluids. Say, "Place rose quartz [where it hurts] and in the heart chakra."

# Ruby

*Power*

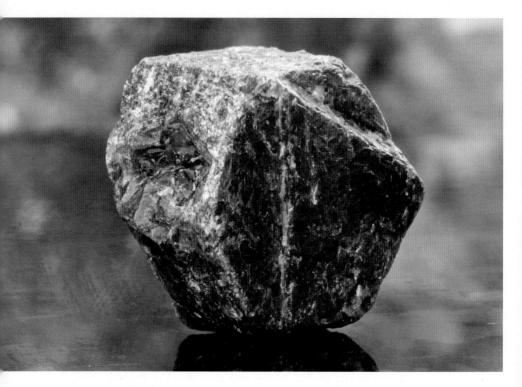

Ruby ethereal crystal stands for power—power in the sense of taking a positive lead with others, success, and taking charge. Taking charge can be in every level of your life. Its vibration brings lushness, wealth, passion, honour, and loyalty.

Ruby energy anchors people to the ground to enjoy all the gorgeousness life on Earth has to offer. So often, as a result of the pain of our life journeys, past lives included, we become scared, distrusting, nervous, and fearful—fearful of receiving all the beauty life offers. Working with ruby energy can help transform this, as it reminds you that you are the creator of your life.

Envelop yourself, body and mind, sky above and earth beneath your feet, with ethereal crystal ruby. This will change the vibration and support you in reconnecting with trust, confidence, and a healthy, beating, emotional heart. Ruby vibration can give you an enormous energy boost when feeling low, tired, or lacking willpower.

Physically, this vibration also improves and heals diabetes, cramps, and tiredness. It helps prevent miscarriage (say, "Place ruby in the womb"), and offers particularly good protection of the baby during pregnancy (say, "Place ruby in and around the womb"). Ruby works positively on the organs of conception and helps protect from and heal infections.

Ruby ethereal crystal offers powerful energy, but it is equally supportive when the problem being treated is a surfeit of energy, such as hyperactivity and ADHD. Ruby grounds the excess energy, allowing the person to drop into their body, feel more grounded, and feel more peaceful and calm.

Finally, when you're working on your money energy and growing your family, surround yourself with the energy of ruby.

# Smoky Quartz

## *Clarity*

Smoky quartz energy is perfect for those of us who have been lied to, as it helps lift the veil so we can see what is real. It is for those who have had enough of living a life obscured by fog. This powerful vibration also supports those who have lived previous lives or current lives as professors, teachers, or enlightened people desperate for and fully involved in awakening people from their "sleep". This ethereal crystal is for people who want to shut down propaganda and make sure that the truth reaches people's ears.

People who are only just "waking up" to what we really are need extra vibrational support so they can further uncover their true being. Clear quartz energy is often too bright, but the vibration of smoky quartz is perfect for helping lift the mist. Smoky quartz energy helps do just that, whether it is a situation, relationship, consciousness awakening, or the answer to a question.

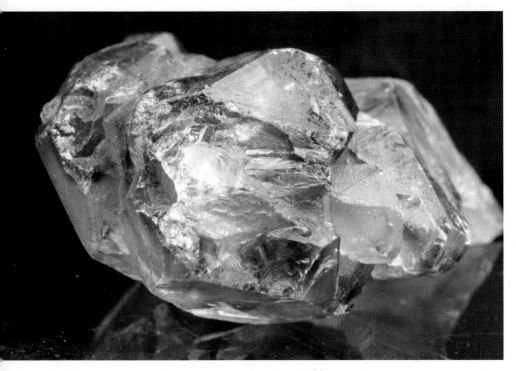

33

As the veil is lifted, smoky quartz energy helps with letting go, opening up, and acceptance, so we can move up to the next level of consciousness and let go of whatever had to go in order to move forward.

Smoky quartz is the ideal ethereal crystal for anyone who has become suspicious and short-sighted because of events in their life. It supports renewed trust and lifts the curtain so we can see clearly and look at our life in peace and beauty. This vibration not only helps unravel the lies of others but also supports us in seeing our own mistakes!

Interesting fact: People who smoke do so out of a desperate need to hide. They are so worried about getting hurt if others see their vulnerability, they hide behind the curtain of smoke from cigarettes, vapes, and cigars. When placing the energy of smoky quartz in the heart, the lungs, on the skin, and in the emotional layer of the aura, this vibration can help someone to quit smoking or at least to smoke a lot less.

As noted, if someone is not ready to use the incredible light of clear quartz, then the energy of smoky quartz is a fantastic ethereal crystal to start with, as it has a beautiful balance between light and earth qualities.

# Sodalite

## *Cosmic Direction*

Sodalite energy is the perfect vibration for seekers, wild souls, and travellers. This ethereal crystal guides you in following your inner voice over mountains and rivers. It is a perfect aid in finding the voice of your intuition. If you have any questions, instead of overthinking and taxing the brain, simply say, "Place sodalite [on this question/situation]." Sodalite leads the way like a babbling brook.

Sodalite has a relaxed vibration and works on all problems linked to a blocked third eye, such as dementia, headaches, eye problems, brain issues, learning difficulties, migraine, obsession, concentration problems, and so on.

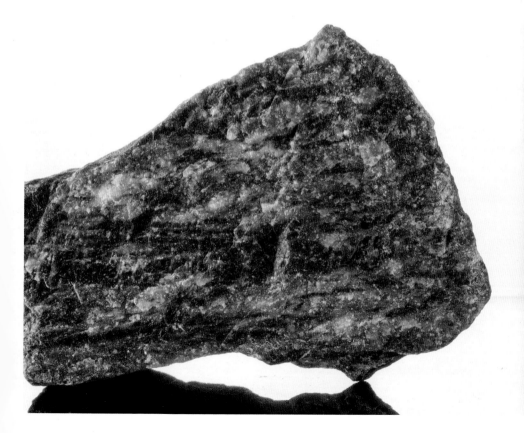

I have noticed in my practice that many problems linked to a blocked third eye have their roots in our previous lives, not this one. The energy of sodalite has a strong healing effect on these problems, as the healing vibrations of ethereal crystals ripple in all directions of time and space, everyone involved. Work with a professional who knows how to cut etheric cords and guide you in Past Life Regression to really heal deeply into this energy point.

When my daughter was born extremely premature, I put the physical crystal sodalite in her sock. She was still tiny and could not kick it off, so it was safe and could not get into her mouth. If you use the physical crystal, always check that they cannot be swallowed and are safe for children when using them! Another reason I now only work with ethereal crystals is that the energy of ethereal crystals can be used on so many diverse levels without ever having to worry about them dislodging, harming, or not being in the right place.

Physically, sodalite helps heal water retention (oedema), helps build the immune system, and makes you very relaxed and content.

# Sphalerite

## *Alignment*

Sphalerite ethereal crystal is an ideal crystal for those who love sports. A divinely perfect, powerful, and successful athlete needs constant realignment of the body and mind. That is exactly what sphalerite brings.

Athletes need grounding. If their energy flits about and disappears into thin air, they will literally lose their balance. Sphalerite energy allows an athlete to repeatedly go deep into their body and anchor their physical body. This ethereal crystal offers athletes physical energy and help with recovery from exercise. Place sphalerite vibration in the muscles.

I also like to throw this ethereal crystal in the mix for people who are lacking strong will, sexuality, openness, and creativity. Place sphalerite around you, in the sexual organs, the womb or prostate, the solar plexus, or in the hips to re-channel the energy deep into the body.

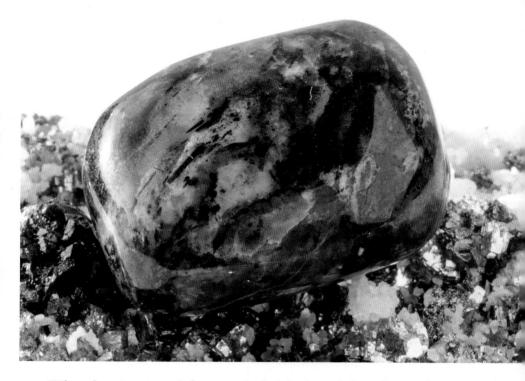

When there is too much focus on the four highest chakras (heart, throat, third eye, and crown), this crystal will help channel energy and put both feet firmly back on the ground. For people who go out of their bodies while meditating, this ethereal crystal will protect and return them to Mother Earth!

Sphalerite realigns energy and gives us back our anchor. You do not need to "fly" to be spiritual; we are in our earthly body and need to respect our earthly connection to be healthy and in balance.

Physically, sphalerite ethereal crystal helps improve the immune system, oxygen intake, aids muscles, heals the reproductive organs, and offers support when there are sexual problems.

Angels who are reincarnated on Earth for the first time tend to want to go back "home". These souls often fear their bodies and their connection with Mother Earth. As a result, many feel depressed, as if they do not belong here. Sphalerite helps them ground and accept their mission on Earth.

# Sunstone

## *Full Circle*

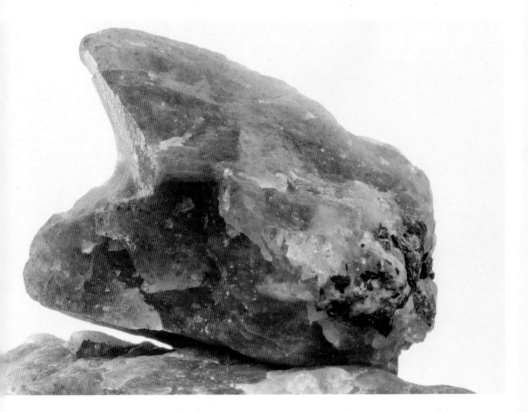

Sunstone energy helps bring a triumphant and successful conclusion to things. It helps people show their feelings without holding back, stands for triumph after a long journey, and supports the creation of something and its desired fruition.

Sunstone creates positivity and gives off light, warmth, and energy to the body and soul. It helps release any issues to do with sexuality, emotions, and creativity. It explicitly helps with the production of breast milk, avoidance of painful menstruation, pregnancy, anaemia, stimulation of the liver and the pancreas, release of back pain, hernia, rheumatism, and building calcium in the body. Sunstone energy strengthens the physical heart and eyes.

You only have to look at what the sun stands for—growth, warmth, and happiness— to know exactly the vibration that sunstone ethereal crystal brings. Working with sunstone when depressed or down helps lift the emotions. If you feel agitated or unsettled, sunstone will change your vibration from fast and rigid to smooth, warm, and full, improving your energy and making you feel calm and trusting.

# Tiger Eye
## *Africa*

When it comes to Tiger Eye energy, think protective voodoo. Tiger eye is extremely powerful if you are in need of protection and to cut jealousy out of your life. Tiger eye sees everything. Nothing can escape from its encapsulating vibration. Tiger eye protects home, body, aura, and mind with heart and soul.

Tiger eye energy warms you up when you are feeling empty and cold inside and breaks the curse of returning patterns of loneliness and heartbreak.

Physically, it helps heal back problems, backache, belly cramps, issues with bones and joints, hernia problems, and protects the baby during pregnancy. It stimulates the liver and pancreas, works positively on the nervous system and has a positive effect on hyperventilation. When struggling with issues of the stomach, liver, intestines, digestive system, or muscles, place tiger eye vibration exactly where needed.

When suffering from acute bronchitis, say, "Place tiger eye in the solar plexus, heart chakra, and bronchi."

Tiger Eye helps heal breathing problems and asthma. When experiencing any type of breathing issues, the person suffering is in a vibration of not taking in the happiness of life. By tuning into the vibration of tiger eye, they will draw in warmth, enjoyment, laughter, and protection of that happiness. Slowly but surely, their life can transform.

Tiger Eye is all about mamas. This is a super vibration to connect with, place around, or anywhere needed when someone wants to be

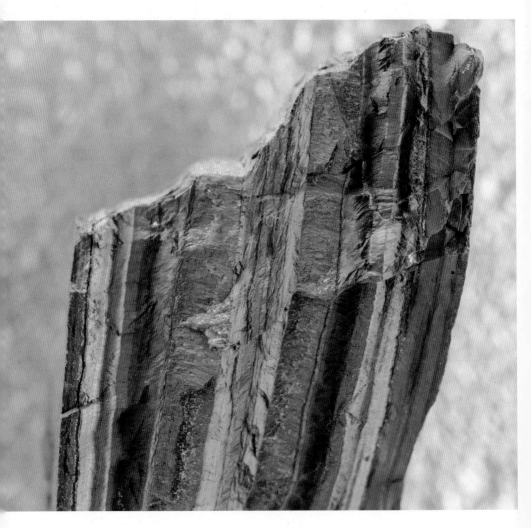

a mother, whether that is becoming a biological mother or through adoption.

If you wish for a baby/child, call in tiger eye and visualize your baby in your arms. Place tiger eye in and around your womb, and visualize preparing your womb as the softest, most cosy, high-vibrational home for your baby.

If you experience difficulties getting pregnant due to hormonal problems or stress, place tiger eye ethereal crystal in the endocrine and nervous systems and the womb or prostate. Tiger eye also helps with milk production.

# Topaz

## *The Path to Success*

Topaz is for those suffering from trauma, and hurt children wishing to be released from childhood to live powerfully and happily as adults. This ethereal crystal helps find the way.

It is nearly impossible for unhealed parents to guide their own children. But for every negative there is a positive, and thanks to those unhealed parents, traumatized children are given a huge opportunity to dig deep within themselves and find the guidance on their own.

We're talking about children growing up with narcissistic parents, victimized parents, alcoholic families, drug-abused families, and families where there has been emotional, physical, or psychological violence.

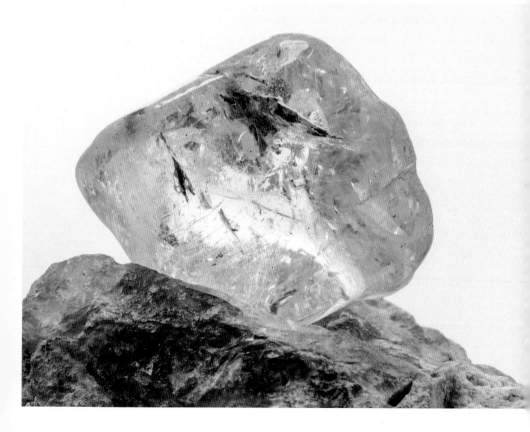

As children, they had to survive by making themselves disappear, and constantly check in with themselves to see whether they were safe or not. Topaz energy gives incredible light to that inner child to help them accept the parents/carers for who they are.

Contrary to popular belief, traumatized children do not need to forgive their parents. If children forgive their parents, then ego stands above them, and children do not ever stand above their parents. What is needed is to accept the parents for who they are and the lessons they brought, and to accept that they acted and were who they were because of their knowledge and consciousness. Be grateful for the biggest gift anyone could have ever given you: life.

This powerful guiding topaz vibration helps you trust your inner knowledge and wisdom and offers gentle spiritual development. The more an individual advances spiritually, the more they can see "the past" for what it was/is and the more the hurt inner child can grow into a wise, understanding, giving and receiving adult. Topaz vibration offers happiness, openness, honesty, and truth to the self.

Say, "Place topaz in the solar plexus", "Place topaz in the heart", "Place topaz in the mind", or "Place topaz on the inner child." Place topaz on childhood memories, past lives, emotions, and connections between the child and the parents to heal the path, soul contracts, and karmic relationships.

Ethereal crystal topaz balances the meridians and stimulates artistic creativity. Meridians are channels through which energy flows throughout the body. They can become blocked by illness, stress, or poor lifestyle choices. The core energy of the flow of the meridians starts in the solar plexus, where the stomach is. When energy flows equally throughout the body, artistic creativity can also flow freely. For anyone who wants more artistic creativity, topaz can be placed in the solar plexus, so you act positively from that inner lead or on the meridians to get the flow going. Topaz can also be placed around the artist or their artist studio for more artistic and creative vibes and connection. Say, "Place topaz in the solar plexus and all the meridians", or "Place topaz on the meridians." Trust that the Universe knows where that is.

Topaz energy has a positive effect on the digestive system, as it stimulates metabolism and taste. It also has a positive influence on anorexia and bulimia. Anorexia is a hugely dangerous mental state caused by literally trying to remove yourself from life, become invisible, removed from every picture of life due to ancestral self-hatred. Topaz energy can help restore energy flow and balance in such situations.

# Tourmaline

## *Protection*

Tourmaline energy is here for those who are fearful—those sensitive souls who struggle with the fast pace of evolution. They have gone through so much at a lower level of consciousness during their past lives they just want to sit in a bubble in this one. Tourmaline conveys the message that you don't need protection because you are always protected.

By placing the energy of tourmaline in the mind, it helps heal the mindset we've had enough of, and as that vibration lifts, new energy is created and we feel and think and know that we are safe, always. We then experience that in our physical life, and things shift so that a brand new, safe environment surrounds us.

Tourmaline energy protects us from the negative thoughts of others (by placing it around the head or in the mind). Sometimes, you may find yourself spiralling into darkness and fear after being out for the day and have no idea how you got there. Most likely, you will have picked up on negative vibrations from the thoughts of others and allowed them in. The higher your vibration, the less likely that is to happen, as like attracts like. Tourmaline energy will help the individual on the journey of lifting thought vibrations. In this way, other people's lower vibrational thoughts won't affect you anymore or you will be able to shift them more easily.

Tourmaline also protects from negative body energies from other people (by placing the energy in your aura). People wash their body so they are clean and smell nice. It's a no-brainer. Why then do people allow dirt from life and others to enter the energy field but never wash it off?

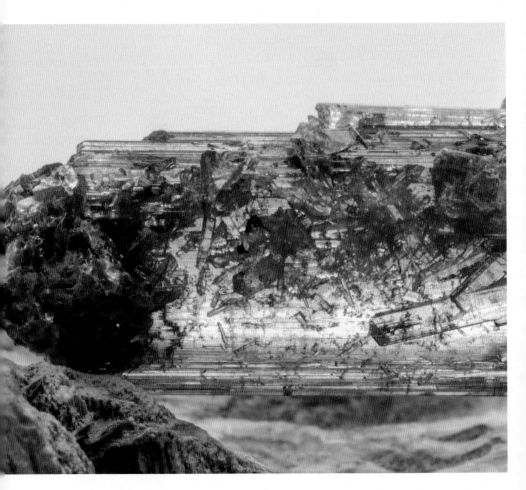

Lower vibrations/dirt from life and others cake together in the energy field and mind and, if not washed off, will negatively affect physical, mental, and emotional health. This can be cleansed with tourmaline energy and prevented from piling up by placing tourmaline ethereal crystal in the aura at the beginning of each day.

When placed around an electrical appliance it keeps the electromagnetic waves local, so it is less tiring and does not have an influence on people. Say, "Place tourmaline around the [phone/TV/laptop, etc.]."

Tourmaline helps us "see the forest for the trees", un-muddle, and take stock of the big picture and not just get caught up in details. In this way, you see where your energy starts and ends and what isn't yours to carry.

In this book, I refer to black tourmaline, but I need to point out that there are other coloured tourmalines in physical form: brown-yellow, blue, green, pink, and a combination of pink and green called watermelon tourmaline. When working with ethereal crystals any colour is possible.

Pink tourmaline offers deep healing but is gentler and "lighter" than black tourmaline. Use blue tourmaline when you're healing and creating on the level of communication and psychic, mental, and love protection. It helps with focus and opens the mind and makes it stronger. It changes negative thoughts into positives, helps with dizzy spells, mental imbalance, and helps overactive and chaotic people centre themselves.

Work with brown or black tourmaline for earthly protection, and physical protection. Tourmaline helps with walking upright, so it is a perfect energy to place in older people's legs, as it literally keeps older people on their feet and protects against physical imbalance.

Tourmaline brings joy in life, confidence, relaxation when nervous, grounding, and calmness. It changes anger and aggression into a positive view of life and gives comfort when sad.

# Turquoise

## *Angelic Guidance*

Turquoise vibration is for people who have had others repeatedly ignore their boundaries, as it helps to clearly set boundaries. It carries the angelic message that we are always guided and protected and communicates to others, "Stop! This is my boundary."

Turquoise is a magical and gentle ethereal crystal. Its warm, kind vibration works as a protector on every level. Travellers should place this vibration around themselves, the plane, the train, the bus, or whatever vehicle they travel in. Motorists especially should place turquoise energy in and around their car before getting on the road.

Turquoise's most important role is to help us distinguish between good and bad. It teaches us to intuit whether someone or something means well or not. It reminds us to work with our intuition and that we can trust and follow it.

Turquoise protects us from rheumatism, joint problems, and issues with blood flow. It reduces pain and minimizes hot flashes during menopause and has a positive effect on everything connected to the liver and cramps.

People who allow their emotions to fester run the risk of eventually manifesting life-threatening illnesses. In particular, those who develop cancer often let others repeatedly breach the healthy boundaries they have set. It is as if other people continually empty their rubbish bins or portable toilets in the person's energy field.

Most of us wouldn't think of not flushing the toilet or not having our rubbish collected and disposed of regularly, yet we allow others to dump their poop in our energy field. If we left our rubbish outside our house, it would be crawling with vermin and mould and smell and rot in no time. That is exactly what happens inside the body when we do not set

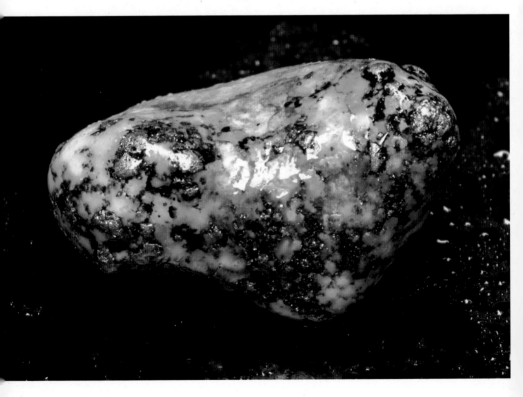

healthy boundaries—first vibrationally, then energetically, and eventually manifested physically as cancer or some other life-threatening illness.

Turquoise ethereal crystal is available to help you set boundaries, protect your energy, digest unresolved emotions, and heal the physical body from cancer if it has come that far in the manifestation process. It also protects against nightmares and prostate disease.

# Unakite

## *Liberation*

We are all connected. The energy contained within our family tree continues, whether we like it or not. Thoughts, emotions, behaviours, good and bad luck—it all continues down the family line. Sometimes it becomes so heavy, it manifests physically in our babies and children as serious issues.

The good thing is that every child born within a certain family line chose that vibration in order to learn lessons and break patterns, grow consciousness, and change the vibration of that family line. It is of course always a mystery as to which of us will be the one to be evolved enough to see the patterns and finally break them. When that happens, liberation is created within the family energy.

The message that unakite brings is liberation from family patterns, behavioural patterns, and all repetitive emotional and thinking patterns. Unakite energy offers radical change, a dramatic cutting of cords, now, in all directions of time and space, everyone involved. Its vibration is here for awakened family members, those waking up and smelling the coffee, who opened their eyes and recognized repetitive patterns, who realize that it will continue unless they break the patterns.

By changing the vibration of repetitive patterns, we stimulate mental growth, raise consciousness, stimulate a higher vibration, and create a new physical experience for everyone involved.

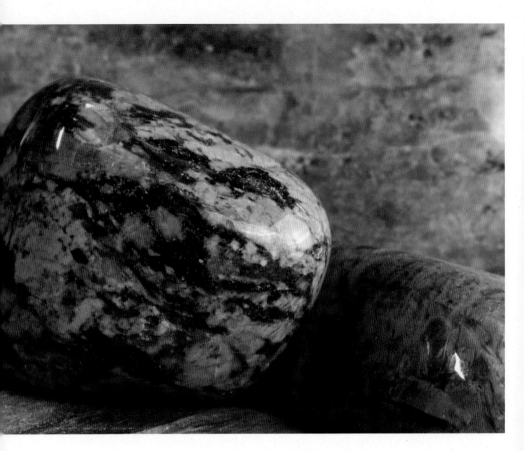

Unakite is an ethereal crystal of the heart. For example, when fears have developed due to problems in love, leading to stubborn, repetitive thoughts and behavioural patterns. Unakite helps restore faith and love in ourselves so that fears disappear and thinking and behavioural patterns change.

Physically, unakite helps restore health and strength after disease or injury. It has a positive effect on sex hormones, protects the health of the baby during pregnancy, supports weight gain when needed, and helps stimulate hair growth.

**Part Three**

# Healing with Ethereal Crystals

# 14

# Meditation with the Ethereal Crystals

## Communicating with and Embodying the Wisdom of the Ethereal Crystals

In your mind's eye, picture the Universe. Now travel to its centre. Visualize its unlimited colours, its crystals in all dimensional shapes and sizes—in the infinite experience of time and space, for everything and anything, anyone, everywhere, anywhere.

Allow the energy of the ethereal crystals to enter your body through the top of your head. As it enters your head, it activates your *knowing*. The incoming energy bursts open in the middle of your head, towards your third eye, and activates your *seeing*, opening fully the gateway between the physical and energetic worlds. It is all one. You become the energetic world. You are the energetic world.

Accept now the energy of the ethereal crystals, which sinks into your throat chakra and opens it so it can receive. You receive everything you need from the ethereal crystals. You receive everything you desire from the ethereal crystals. You ask and you are given, in all directions of time and space everyone involved, now.

Allow the energy to fill your heart and take on the shape of a diamond. Accept the diamond of Brahman. Say to yourself, "My deepest truth, and that of others, connects with my heart, now and always—perfect health, love, and abundance."

Feel the unconditional love from the energy of the diamond, which contains the energy of all the ethereal crystals. Feel perfect health. Feel perfect happiness. Now let that vibration radiate into your whole being.

Take a deep breath in, then breathe out.

Now see the energy of the ethereal crystals continuing to fill your body, moving into your solar plexus, where your stomach is. Allow yourself to act fully from a place of acceptance, love, and trust in the ethereal crystals, for the goodness of humanity and beyond.

Now allow the energy of the ethereal crystals to fill your cauldron, that magical place inside our bellies that is linked to magical creation: your pelvis, hips, womb, and ovaries, if you are a woman, or your prostate if you are a man. Say to yourself, "I am the creation of life. I create for myself and others in divine perfection, through a knowing, receiving, loving, and positive action."

Now, using the ethereal crystals, create a new, exciting, miraculous, out-of-this-world, life. Allow the vibrations to be received in the deepest parts of your cells, in your cauldron, in all directions of time and space.

Now allow the energy of the ethereal crystals to go deeper—into your roots, into the earth, into earthly life, our mirror. Visualize an infinite number of roots spreading into Mother Earth. Visualize their energy, vibrations, colours, and shapes. Visualize healing now. Visualize the crystals inside Mother Earth being activated and renewed. Allow the physical results of energetic knowing, seeing, receiving, acting, and creativity to become physical—perfect health, love, happiness, and abundance.

Take a deep breath in, and breathe out.

When you're ready, bring your attention back to your heart, and visualize the energy of all of those beautiful ethereal crystals starting to vibrate far beyond the boundaries of your physical body. It becomes everything, all at once. Know that all you need to do is ask for what you want, and in a snap of the fingers it is there, as the vibrations of the ethereal crystals are already in you.

Now bring your attention to your crown chakra on top of your head. Visualize two pyramids intertwined, one pointing up, and one pointing down, like a hexagram. Accept the perfect state of balance achieved between man and the Universe. Align these two intertwined pyramids with the energy of your heart chakra and your root chakra, where your coccyx is.

Now, as you breathe in and out, free yourself from the boundaries of the earthly world and its limitations, so all that remains is just you and the ethereal crystals, in perfect health, love, happiness, and abundance. You stand in the midst of the ethereal crystals, one with the all-encompassing energy of all that is. Receive, create, and give, in divinely perfect balance. Allow it, and accept it now.

# 15

# Improving Your State of Mind with Ethereal Crystals

## Healing your Consciousness Using Ethereal Crystals

Our conscious mind involves our daily thoughts, and its vibrational home is in and around the head. Everything we experience, see, hear, feel, believe, and think in life we do with the conscious mind. From there, everything is sent through to the subconscious mind and on to the Universe, where what we believe and feel become programmed habits, thoughts, and emotions.

Energetically, the conscious and subconscious minds overlap. The conscious mind is the signpost that points the way to the subconscious mind, and back again to the conscious mind, like a boomerang returning the same vibrational things we believe, feel, and think.

In turn, we send this vibration out into the world, and it becomes a physical reality. Lower vibrations of fear, pain, and shame create the physical experiences of those vibrations and continue to do so until we consciously change things. Higher vibrations of happiness, love, and abundance create the physical experience of those same vibrations.

During the process of changing the vibration in our conscious thinking, we change how we think and feel, thereby signposting new energy into our subconscious mind, which makes us feel better, think more positively, and change what the boomerang brings back to us. It is not just ourselves we are healing. By healing ourselves and becoming more positive in our outlook, we heighten the vibrations of the collective consciousness, too. We are all one.

Until the age of seven, we are all somewhat hypnotized by the vibrations (emotions and beliefs) of our family, carers, friends, and others around us. We are programmed to experience certain vibrations from a very young age. When you become conscious of where certain fears, thoughts, emotions come from, you may start to realize they were never yours to begin with, but belonged to your mother, father, grandmother, or someone else. Because you witnessed and were surrounded by that person's energy all the time, you took it on as your own.

You don't need to know where your lower vibration comes from. You can simply place the high vibration of ethereal crystals in your subconscious mind, your emotions, your fears, your thinking patterns, and start the transformation process.

Any ethereal crystal can help with this, depending on which one you feel is most appropriate. If you're looking for suggestions, unakite is an excellent choice, as it cuts family, thinking, behavioural, and emotional patterns. Say, "I place unakite on this fear", or "I place unakite in my subconscious mind", or "I place unakite on my family line."

Healing can take place immediately. If it doesn't, remember that humans are creatures of habit—we love going back to what we don't want simply because it's what we know. The fast train between the conscious and subconscious mind is so used to giving and receiving a certain vibration, you will need to be persistent if you want to see a change in what it is used to signposting. Your struggles took time to establish in your vibration; changing them will also take time.

Here are four steps to success:

1 **Be accountable:** You make the decision that change will take place and you are the one doing it. You take full responsibility and positive action.
2 **Recognize patterns:** You see within yourself what's happening. Maybe even write it down. You recognize the patterns of your reactions, actions, thoughts, and emotions.
3 **Change the vibration:** Work with the ethereal crystals to change the vibration.
4 **Be persistent:** It may take time, so keep with it.

You don't build muscle in a day, so stick with it. When you do, change is inevitable. Notice subtle changes, and celebrate them! Celebration and gratitude are high vibrations. The more you notice and feel them, the faster your vibration will rise. As a result, your healing and new-life-creation-process will flow faster and faster.

## Subconscious Mind

Our subconscious mind is powerful, but it obeys the conscious mind. Whatever it is given by the conscious mind, it says, "Okay, here it is." Thus, whatever gets signposted by the conscious mind goes to the subconscious mind and boomerangs back to the conscious mind.

You are a human being with a free will. The subconscious mind says, "Your wish is my command." It can reflect back the deepest low to the highest high. It holds all of the information and knowledge ever accumulated, experienced, seen, felt, and heard. In our subconscious mind, we find our true self—who we are, what we are here for, where we come from—but also everything accumulated in the past from family beliefs to normal life experiences.

The vibrations of our subconscious mind energetically circle around our third eye (between the eyebrows), our crown chakra (top of the head), our eighth chakra (15 cm above the head), and our ninth chakra (30cm above the head) and above. Our family beliefs are found in the lower part of the subconscious mind, around the third eye, crown chakra, and eighth chakra. The higher part of the subconscious mind, around the ninth chakra and above, holds our blueprint; that is, who we really are in absolute perfection and all unlimited possibilities.

You change the way you think and feel by changing the vibration through placing the ethereal crystals directly in the third eye, crown and eighth chakras and unblocking that energy stream, so that the unlimited high energy from the ninth chakra can flow to your conscious mind.

The following story about how ethereal crystals changed the vibration in the collective consciousness is a beautiful example of what can happen when consciously changing vibration. It astonished me then, and still gives me goose bumps when I write about it now.

My husband and I bought our first house together many years ago, south of Belgium. Even though it needed a lot of work, the house was gorgeous: a French château built in 1912. What we didn't know yet was that it was the most expensive house in the poorest village in the country, and thus represented status but amid few resources—my family's vibration.

When the previous owners bought it, it still had guns and hand grenades in the basement left behind by German soldiers during the second world war. The German army had occupied the house, and fierce battles were fought in the area. On our first night there, I had visions of people trying to break in and rob us, a vibration left over from my own family's experiences. A few years later, the house was broken into while we were asleep. It is poignant to realize now that it was a reflection of the vibration I myself was carrying.

There was no work in the area. People died young. Life-threatening illnesses and drug rates were high. In other words, the consciousness was low, and the land was exhausted, resulting in unpleasant and low-vibrational physical experiences. We make subconscious decisions, led by our vibration, as like attracts like.

We lived there for just over five years before we moved back to the UK, where my husband grew up. By then, my two eldest children had learned to speak French, so I decided to keep going back twice a year so they could keep up the French language.

After distancing ourselves from the place, everything had become clear to me, and I started to realize how it all works. I had been guided there originally because my relationship with my husband needed certain lessons and healing on that land, and because it was in my vibration.

Now I needed to heal the general land and consciousness of the people, and by doing so, I healed myself too.

I worked with the following ethereal crystals:

- **Smoky quartz:** Lift the veil and see what is real. This vibration would bring awareness.
- **Amethyst:** Purification
- **Clear quartz:** Pure light

I placed the energy of the ethereal crystals in the ground so they could send out their vibrations for miles, to wherever it was needed, and on the consciousness of the people, to heal them and change the vibration, energy, and physical outcomes. I didn't know what was going to happen; I only knew that the land and collective consciousness needed healing.

A few months later I read in the newspapers that the local police had made one of the country's biggest drug busts—indeed, in all of Europe—in the area! The vibrations of the ethereal crystals had lifted the veil to show what was real. They had purified the land and the people and brought light that pushed out the dark.

As mentioned, I didn't know what the outcome would be, but by working with ethereal crystals, by adding high vibrational healing, I changed the vibration and the energy, which led to the best possible physical outcome. That best possible physical outcome is something you need to trust. Working with ethereal crystals, you will always get what you set out to receive, and better—whether that's a physical result or a feeling.

# 16

# Healing Nature with Ethereal Crystals

## Working with the Energy of Ethereal Crystals to Heal Animals and Nature

Just like everything else on this planet, animals and nature are created as the result of vibration. This means that we can heal, change, and transform life for nature and animals by placing ethereal crystals for healing.

Even though animals have a different consciousness, they too are influenced by their past lives, environment, upbringing, and experiences. They are who they are because of their vibration. They too experience what they experience because of their current vibration. Ethereal crystals can help heal, change, and transform animals' lives.

As we heal Mother Earth, we also heal ourselves, because the planet is a reflection of humanity. Her fire is our anger. Her floods are our undigested emotions. Her tornados and extreme winds are our spinning heads and instability and not knowing what to do any more.

You can place ethereal crystals on forest fires; for example, chrysocolla is a calming vibration. To use it, say, "Place chrysocolla in the ground where the forest fire is. Place chrysocolla on the fire." By changing the vibration, the energy changes and so will the physical outcome. The fire dies down and does not reignite, because everything physical starts with a vibration.

Change the quality of rivers, streams, and oceans by placing ethereal crystals in them. By adding these high vibrations, we can transform the vibrations in the planet's waters. New vibrations in our waters create a new energy, a new flow; one of more oxygen, more happiness, more gorgeousness. The waters flow better and are of higher quality, and this affects the animals in the water and us humans.

We are all one consciousness. Healing the water on the planet affects the human emotions positively.

Place ethereal crystals on groups of animals that are in danger of going extinct, using perhaps citrine or sunstone to go beyond what is. Or place sphalerite ethereal crystal to realign that animal's energy and root them back into the planet. To do this, place ethereal crystals on the consciousness of the animal going extinct.

Placing ethereal crystals in the roots of plants helps them ascend to a whole new level. It will create flora (and fauna) of a whole new dimension, in line with the new Aquarian era we have entered.

Ethereal crystals are easy to use in daily life. Before drinking a glass of water, place the ethereal crystals you feel/know you need in your water. In this way, all the healing vibrations of these ethereal crystals will be taken into the body when drinking that glass of water. Use from one to five ethereal crystals. Place them in your food, on your vegetable garden, on the farm. Use them in your pets' water and on your plants. With one fingersnap, we heal, change, and transform things every day. One drop in a bucket might look like nothing, but continue to add drops every day and you will see big results.

# Saving the World with Ethereal Crystals

## Healing Mother Earth and Improving Life on Earth

The previous chapter is an important part of what I'm sharing here. By healing the planet, we heal ourselves. By healing our waters, we heal our emotions. By healing the forest fires, we heal our anger. By healing storms, we ground ourselves again.

Let's take it a step further. By healing past life energies, by healing everything that has ever happened on Mother Earth, we can let go of old stories and create new ones. We can literally create a whole new planet, consciousness, and experiences. We raise vibration and literally rise and create a completely new world.

Everything that has ever happened on our planet is stored in Mother Earth, just as the emotions connected to all that has happened to us are stored in our physical bodies as vibrations. I'm sure you have been to certain places and felt uncomfortable. Or the opposite has happened: You sit somewhere and don't want to move because it just feels so right! These are vibrations that we feel, memories of the past that we feel, still sending their vibrations out into the world.

Once, we were walking in Cornwall in the southwest of England, and the land was absolutely stunning! It would have been easy to be misled by those gorgeous views, but my intuition told me that this place was still carrying a lot of pain. I received a vision of the earth opening up and hundreds of men dying. I shared this with a local, and he said that this was land where extensive mining had taken place and several catastrophes had occurred there. I had intuited what had happened as these vibrations were still present.

I placed the transformative vibrations of ethereal crystals in the land to remove those memories from Mother Earth and human vibrations, and in this way, healed every person who experienced that tragedy. Even though it was a very long time ago, these souls might have still been carrying that vibration in their reincarnations. By healing the land and the event, it healed all humans involved in all directions of time and space.

As we continued to walk, we came to another beautiful place. Even though it was also stunning, when I tuned into the vibrations there, I could feel a lot of battle and death. Once again, when I asked locally, I was told that the Romans had invaded Britain via the exact same place where we were standing, and these vibrations were still present. So I went ahead and placed a new vibration with ethereal crystals in order to heal those events and all people involved, in all directions of time and space.

The following are some different ways we can change the vibrations of past and current events:

- When we know what has happened in a specific place, we can place crystals in Mother Earth there, either where you're standing or on the other side of the world.
- When we find out about a past life, we can place ethereal crystals on that past life. Say, "Place [name of ethereal crystals] on this past life, its location, and everyone involved."
- When you are feeling that a place doesn't have a high vibration, tune in with your intuition and ask what ethereal crystals it needs, then place them.

# 18

# Cleansing Energy in Buildings

## Making Any Space Feel Comfortable Again

A room feels a certain way depending on its vibration, and that will depend on what has happened there—what has happened on the land where the building is; who has lived, worked, or been there; the words that have been spoken; the actions that have taken place.

That's a lot to take in. But all you need to remember is that by placing the ethereal crystals in line with what vibration you'd like in the space, everything will automatically transform.

Here are some suggestions:

While waiting your turn in the doctor's waiting room, you could place clear quartz (light), agate (healer of everything), smoky quartz (creating insights), watermelon tourmaline (protection), or amethyst (purification). Do the same in supermarkets if it doesn't feel right.

A few years ago, I was waiting for my son to finish his gymnastics class, and the waiting room felt very uncomfortable. I could feel jealousy and rivalry. To counter this, I placed aquamarine (communication), lapis lazuli (friendship), and clear quartz (replacing darkness and heaviness with light and comfortable energies) in the room and could clearly feel the unpleasant vibrations being lifted. The whole atmosphere changed!

When I attend a fair for work, I always check the building before I arrive. Once, a fair took place in a hotel that had previously been a psychiatric hospital. I placed onyx in the building to release the deep pain, amethyst to purify all vibrations, and smoky quartz so that any spirits stuck there would lift the veil and see that it was time to return home to the light.

When visiting anyone in hospital, before going in, I place clear quartz and amethyst in the building to clear and cleanse it and raise the awareness of the patients, medical staff, and visitors. Doing this helps everyone expand their consciousness and realize that they are the creators of their own physical health. Also feel what else the building needs and place it in or around the space. For example, place turquoise in your aura as protection before entering a hospital, along with any other ethereal crystal you think is needed.

One day during my hospital stay with my 1lb baby, another baby that was a few weeks old was brought into the Neonatal Intensive Care Unit as he wasn't breathing. They did everything they could to save him, but I could "see" that he had already crossed over when they brought him in. A day later, they decided to turn off his life support.

I was staying at the hospital at that time to be close to my baby as I lived two hours away, and the staff asked me to change room. This was clearly organized by the Universe. The hospital staff asked me to move into the room where the parents of the little boy who had passed away stayed, and the second I opened the door, the energy plummeted. The room was filled with pain and grief.

At first, I felt slightly annoyed with my guides, thinking: *Hang on. I'm going through a tough time here and am focused on my daughter, and now I have to sort this energy out, too?* Of course, I did sort it out. I couldn't enter the room as the energy was too painful, so I did this healing.

I imagined a tornado tearing through the room, picking up all the lower vibrations. I placed four suction pipes on the corners of the room and then guided the tornado to one of the corners and saw everything sucked away instantly into Mother Earth. I saw all the leftover lower vibrations with my mind's eye, then sucked them towards other corners until they were all gone. I then filled the room with green-coloured light, which I had explode. Next, I washed my hands to cleanse of any potential energy debris. When I returned half an hour later, the room was cleared. In this case I used shapes to change the energy.

# Healing Human Connections

## Improving Relationships by Working with Ethereal Crystals

When relationships with certain people are difficult, unfriendly, or tiring, say, "Place [name of the ethereal crystal] on the connection between me and [first name of the other person]." Give yourself a minute, breathe in calmly, and feel how the changes occur.

You may experience a shiver or twitch of the body as the negative connection and energies are released. It's nothing to worry about, because good vibes and connections can never be broken. If you do ethereal crystal healing with the intention of making things better, it always ripples out in all directions of time and space, for the highest good of everyone concerned.

As noted earlier, we often experience our lives according to the vibrations of our parents before we realize that can be changed.

People sometimes say, "It's in my genes."

To which I answer, "So don't turn them on."

We are all vibration, and it is up to you whether you turn it on, make it stronger, and continue the vibration. Everything a biological mother fears, believes, thinks, and feels at the time of birth settles in the new baby's vibration as they come into the world. No baby is born with a clean slate. We are energy, all connected.

When we want to change, leave our childhood behind, live differently from our family, we need to start by removing the mother's energy from our energy system. By placing ethereal crystals on that connection, we can start to change these vibrations. In this way, you set yourself free and heal your whole female line.

If there are specific issues, such as fertility problems, fear of creating new life, emotional roller-coasters, or sexual issues, place ethereal crystals specifically on the connection, belly to belly, between partners. If there are specific issues linked to grief or sadness, place ethereal crystal healing specifically between the hearts of mother and child. Follow your intuition with this.

This can also be done for the father's line, or for other relationships. No matter what you're struggling with, a person can be transformed.

For example, let's say that you struggle with trust. This lack of trust most likely because you experienced relationships and encounters where trust was broken. It could be that you don't necessarily know where the trust issues are coming from. To work with this, say, "Place [your chosen ethereal crystals] on all relationships in all directions of time and space linked to trust issues." The Universe will know exactly where those vibrations need healing.

Energy is passed on from parents to children. I call them Family Energy Circles. People say they have a hereditary illness. Nothing is "hereditary"; everything is energy. It is only hereditary because we believe it is. Vibration is passed on from parent to child, and sometimes, it is the child who pays for it when the energy gets clogged and they are the first to experience physical issues. This is obviously nothing to feel guilty about, because it is part of life and awareness.

Let me give an example from my own experience to make this clear.

While I was spending time on the Neonatal Intensive Care Unit with my extremely premature baby girl, I felt this heavy energy around a baby boy there. He had become distressed in the womb, defecated in his own amniotic fluid, and started breathing it in. This had damaged his lungs, and potentially also his brain. Following the birth, he was having severe problems.

I sat in my room, pictured the baby boy in my imagination, and did the work.

As I asked the Universe if there was anything else, it was made clear to me that a family circle coming from the father's side was at the root of

148

the problem. (I can't stress enough that this all happens subconsciously, and there is nothing to feel guilty about.)

I could see a blanket of emotional problems now lying on the child and coming from the father. I placed ethereal crystals between them and watched as all that energy moved back to the father, away from the baby. I could see energetically that the father started crying uncontrollably when his emotional baggage returned to him. Because the father's emotional baggage was no longer with his son, the baby's vibration could rise and the physical issues he was dealing with no longer matched that vibration, which meant that the child could heal. He lit up and now had a very shiny presence, clearly happy that this burden had been lifted from him.

I could now see that that vibration came from the father's mother, so I helped him to energetically give it back to *his* mother as I placed ethereal crystals for healing. Whatever was left with him I surrounded with the colour green, so that he would heal this and do the same with his mother, the baby's grandmother.

I later heard from the baby's mother, whom I met regularly in the parents' room, that her baby boy was progressing well and the doctors were hopeful. I could feel that he was going to be fine.

In my twenties and early thirties, I struggled with PMS, mood swings, and postnatal depression. When I analyze myself and my family, I finally understand why I felt the way I did. Through past life regression therapy, I experienced the many lives of emotional manipulation and suppression I had gone through and the vibration I carried from those times. I always felt as though I wasn't allowed to be who I am.

On top of that, I was carrying family circle vibrations with me, which I alluded to earlier. My father's side observed strict religious prohibitions on lust and emotional manipulation, and signs of excess alcohol use began to show up in the family. These conditions settle in the root (first) and sacral (second) chakras and represent the right to be and the right to feel. My mother's side was ruled by heavy vibrations of guilt and shame, dating back to vibrations that became seriously stuck in the relationship between my great-grandmother and my grandfather, leading to a love-hate relationship and feelings of rejection.

In addition to this energetic burden from the past, I suffered a huge amount of stress as a young child when my parents went through a divorce. The relationship with my first stepmother was far from an enjoyable one, and stress levels and emotions ran high for me, starting from the age of five.

It is this energy that led to my daughter's extreme premature birth, as I recounted earlier, and I had a streptococcus A infection in my womb, which nearly killed my baby and me a few days after she was born. Fortunately, what could have been my deepest low became my greatest awareness opener, and I started to heal and change.

I placed ethereal crystals on all those connections, people alive and dead, to change those vibrations. I unclogged that energy by changing vibration, as it was my decision to live differently. And as I changed all those vibrations, I transformed my thinking, emotions, and life. We are all connected, and there is only the now. My healing transcended all directions of time and space, everyone involved. And with my healing, I broke the vibrations within my family circles.

# Healing of Situations

## Healing Past and Present Situations so that New Opportunities Can Arise

When something happens, we can feel pretty shaken and uncomfortable. We get focused on the subject, think more dark and negative thoughts, and before we know it, we are stuck in a negative circle. Low emotions and thoughts are pumped into our subconscious mind, which obeys and gives back more.

Before we know it, we think that's who we are: negative thinkers and depressed, anxious people, lowering our vibration. The thing is, we're not; we just allowed the conscious mind to take control, instead of taking control ourselves.

Start by breathing from the belly into the heart, deeply and calmly, until you feel the benefit of it. Next, decide which ethereal crystals each person needs and which ethereal crystals the situation needs. Picture the situation in your mind, along with everyone involved.

As you picture this, take a moment to see what happens when you talk, listen, and interact with each mentally. See in your mind's eye who stands where and how people and the situation are presented to you, as that will give you additional information.

If you struggle to see the situation, no worries; it's all in the intention. Use your intention to place ethereal crystals on the people involved and the connection between you. Observe these connections however they present themselves to you—they can simply consist of the space between you and someone else.

Once you've placed the ethereal crystals, you might notice that, thanks to the healing vibrations, the situation suddenly starts to unfold differently. Time is linear; everything happens now. If you rewrite a situation with healing, that first lower-energy situation no longer has any influence over you.

Once you realize this, breathe calmly and relax. See or feel or simply know that everything is settling down and the event and connection to other people is being healed.

When you are ready, let it go—perhaps see it fly away in a hot-air balloon—and come back to the here and now.

Sometimes, words are uttered during arguments that really don't help the situation. Words have an incredibly strong effect, and their vibration ripples out. When situations need healing, words may also need to be healed. Please be careful to choose your words carefully.

When low-vibrational words are used, you can undo their unpleasant energy by placing an ethereal crystal on them. The best one to use is clear quartz, because it gives so much light it overpowers the darkness of the words. In your mind, say, "Place clear quartz on those words."

I once visited a holy site in Belgium with a friend and one of my sisters. I desperately tried to enjoy it, but something felt off. It had a statue of Mother Mary, where people came for healing, and that felt lovely, but everywhere else, including in the surrounding woods, I found myself struggling. There was a big, old building on the site, and I thought I saw a stern, older man peeping through the window and staring at us. I felt haunted, watched, and hurt.

After leaving the site, my friend asked us about our experience at the site, and we quickly found out that we had all experienced the same feeling. We found out that a long time ago, the building next to the site had been a school for orphans run by Catholic priests, and I don't think the priests had been very nice to the pupils.

I decided to address this by placing ethereal crystal healing on any potential negative events that had occurred at the site, as well as on the building and grounds. This healed and changed the vibrations in all directions of time and space, everyone involved.

A client of mine had been pregnant but lost the baby at 20 weeks. She then suffered several further miscarriages before, thankfully, she became pregnant again. This time, she carried the child to term but now had gone over her due date and came to see me.

Tragedies such as those this woman had suffered with her earlier pregnancies leave deep energetic scars in the womb, ovaries, hips, emotions, and heart, and I could feel that she was subconsciously holding him in to keep him safe in her belly. Unfortunately, because she was overdue, she risked needing a Caesarean section, which she really didn't want. I could feel that the baby was also holding back, as he was immersed in the vibration of fear created by the heartache the mother had experienced with the loss of her other babies.

I told her that I could feel that the vibrations from the other baby and miscarriages were still present in her womb, and what she could do was simply talk to her baby about how excited she was to meet him and how it was safe to be born. I also placed ethereal crystals in her womb and removed the heartbreaking energy of the past pregnancies, otherwise the new baby would be born with those vibrations of fear and a broken heart. That evening, she went into labour and delivered a healthy baby boy into this world.

# Healing the Physical Body

## Improving and Healing Physical Disease with Ethereal Crystals

### Healing and Strengthening Blood

After giving blood, add ethereal crystals to the bag to potentize the donated blood and send beautiful vibrations to the recipient. Say, "Place clear quartz, hematite, and fluorite in the blood", and point to the blood bag physically or in your mind.

Why clear quartz? Its light is so bright and cleansing, it heals anything.

Why hematite? This is *the* blood stone. It helps with anaemia, physical weakness, courage, strength, and homeostasis.

Why fluorite? This stone is a motivational one, and offers physical and spiritual energy. Many life-threatening diseases have their roots in blocked higher chakras. Fluorite is ideal for unblocking these higher chakras and healing disease. It also is a support when undergoing major operations, and works positively on bone marrow, cells, and diseases such as leukaemia and other cancers. Fluorite is the crystal of re-birth and transformation. Working with its frequency can help by literally giving new life.

### Cure Your Blood

When coming off painkillers or other drugs, place hematite in the blood to prevent pain after the drugs leave the body. The vibration of hematite allows blood to be rejuvenated and strengthened.

## Unblocking the Bowels

For help with constipation and difficulty defecating, place tiger eye and rose quartz in the intestines. Issues with opening the bowels are mental and emotional and indicate a problem in letting go.

## Healing Physical Wounds, Pain, and Other Problems

If a child falls and cuts their knee, place amethyst on the wound as it works wonders on the skin. If you pull a muscle, place sphalerite in the muscle.

For back pain, let me share what worked for me in the following story.

Overnight, I had developed serious back spasms and could hardly walk or move. Back pain occurs when there are problems in your mind related to the support you are receiving in your life. Pain in the mid back is specifically related to not feeling supported in the actions you want to take in life, and I clearly needed to feel more support.

When I was still experiencing back pain two days later, I turned to ethereal crystals for support. I placed sunstone, citrine, and onyx on my back muscles. Sunstone and citrine give off pure light and happiness, and onyx would help heal the vibration of grief stuck in my back from not feeling supported in my life. I placed amethyst in my spine to open my consciousness and allow me to realize what was going on with my back so it could be dealt with and helped to heal. Finally, I placed soda-lite and moonstone in the tissue around the spine to calm and heal old emotional vibrations that had settled in my back tissue.

An hour after doing this, my back pain was much reduced, and by the next day, it was as good as gone.

## Healing Serious Physical Illnesses and Problems such as Allergies

As I explained earlier, every disease, illness, or health problem is just a vibration that can be changed, and as a result, no problem or disease is easier or more difficult to cure.

It may be true that cancer involves a deeper energetic imbalance, but it can be as easy to transform as any other disease. It is all about trust; that is, the belief that our natural state is perfect health, and that the Universe has power beyond limits and is present in the vibrations of the ethereal crystals, as well as in us.

When it comes to treating allergies, one approach that has not yet been explored is, you guessed it, working to address our vibrational levels. At the end of the day, every physical disease has vibrational roots created by an emotion caused by an experience. So let's look at allergies and the many ways we are "allergic" to life situations.

During the last 20 years, people have become more stressed for a variety of reasons. They may have a job to which they are literally "allergic" but keep doing it out of fear of not finding anything else, not being able to pay the mortgage, and so on, and end up in an allergic-to-the-job downward spiral. Or perhaps we socialize because we "have to" in order to maintain social status, when we are actually allergic to socializing in that way and would far prefer to be at home relaxing in the garden.

In short, people may be allergic to people and situations in their lives. So, to what or to whom are you really allergic?

We have lived so many lives before this one, and we are who we are because of the things we have been through in our past lives. Unless you heal and cleanse those past vibrations, they are still present in you, in both your subconscious and conscious mind. Why? Because time is linear; everything happens in the here and now.

History teaches us that our level of consciousness and awareness were nowhere near what they are today in earlier times, due to war, cruelty, nastiness, pain, and poverty. We were literally allergic to the awful house we lived in, losing loved ones because there was no medical care, allergic to selfish kings and lords and masters, allergic to extremely low-paid jobs and abuse at work. The list goes on. You may not consciously remember this, but unless you're a reincarnated angel, you have been through it, and it is still present in your vibration.

Allergies from birth (I always talk about past lives and the present one) may be associated with the following specific body parts:

**Coccyx:** To do with earthly fears. Think of the past centuries, with their lies, deceit, rape, violence, stealing, loss, dirt, and hunger, all of which lead to confidence and trust issues. You have created an allergy against those happenings and people still present in your energy system.

**Heart:** To do with repressed desires that lead to embarrassment and sadness. Your heart carries the vibration of balance and love. Are you in balance? Is your heart open to love and to being loved? Past lives and the current life events have made us close our hearts out of fear due to events and other people. You have become allergic to beautiful earthly things because life on Earth has caused you so much harm and heartache.

**Head:** To do with withheld information, education that suppresses curiosity, invalidation of beliefs, no right to ask anything or think for yourself, lies, misinformation, spiritual abuse, deep-seated feelings, and not having dealt with events. These situations are similar to the ones involving the coccyx that have made you allergic to certain situations and people due to anger, fear, and despair. They are still carried in your vibration, and that eventually comes out as physical disease or in this case, allergies.

Note: People allergic to tree, grass, and flower pollen and to certain foods have gone through such trauma during past lives or in this one they have literally become allergic to things belonging to life on Earth. People who suddenly have an allergic reaction later in life (not from birth) are most likely reacting to something that happened in this life.

## How Can Ethereal Crystals Heal Allergies?

To help heal allergies, I would place ethereal crystals in the coccyx, blood, heart, head, and other places on the body showing symptoms, such as the eyes, lungs, airways, throat, skin, and all of the connections to the cause of the allergies. The following is a list of suggested ethereal crystals to assist you:

- Coccyx – Jasper, and/or black tourmaline, and/or onyx
- Blood – Morganite
- Heart – Morganite, and/or unakite, and/or onyx, and/or green tourmaline
- Head – Fluorite and/or sodalite
- Skin – Green amethyst, and/or purple amethyst, and/or onyx, and/or green aventurine
- Symptoms: Chrysocolla, and/or amber, and/or agate, and/or aquamarine
- Connections to the cause: Morganite, and/or unakite, and/or watermelon tourmaline, and/or turquoise, and/or smoky quartz, and/or clear quartz

Note: As always, feel free to ignore the above suggestions and decide for yourself which ethereal crystals are best for you.

Here are the specific steps to follow:

- Check out which ethereal crystals your aura and mind need.
- Place the ethereal crystals by intention—I recommend the following schedule:
- Every morning for five days, followed by two days of rest, then:
- One further day placing ethereal crystals
- One week later another placing of ethereal crystals
- One week later another placing of ethereal crystals
- After that monthly placings, or keep going weekly for a bit longer. Listen to your intuition.

## Child with Conjunctivitis

Here is an example of healing I carried out on my daughter who developed conjunctivitis.

First, I placed blue lace agate ethereal crystal in her eyes using my intention as it is good for children and wards off infections and colds. I said, "Place blue lace agate in the eyes of [first name]."

Then I placed amethyst on her eyes, as it works wonders on the eyes and is ideal for cleansing. I said, "Place amethyst on the eyes of [name]."

I placed the ethereal crystals with strong loving intention. I knew the vibrational change was happening and repeatedly said out loud, "Our natural state is perfect health."

After a little giggle, because she found all this very funny, she went to sleep for the night.

The next morning, her eyes showed signs of healing. The stickiness had gone and only a little redness remained. A small amount of stickiness came back, but I trusted the healing, and two days later her eyes returned to their natural state of health.

## Child with Sty

The next example shows that this healing method can be done wherever you are.

We were in a café in a sports complex when my son said his eye was hurting. When I looked, I saw a sty between his eyelashes at the bottom of his eye. He wanted me to put some "stones" on it to make it go away. His belief was already there, which really helped. He knew that if Mum puts stones on it, it will go away.

I said, "Place amethyst on the sty of [first name]." Amethyst is the perfect stone for cleansing and eyes.

By the evening it was fading and the next day, the sty was gone.

## Extremely Premature Baby

Because my youngest daughter was born 16 weeks premature, the doctors labelled her as having "chronic lung disease". They saw a baby born with huge lung issues and expected continued issues as a result. As I said earlier, that went in one ear and out the other. From the beginning, I changed her path by changing her vibration.

During her first winter in nursery, she started to cough heavily. My gut instinct said it was nothing to worry about, but I went to see the doctor for confirmation. Before I took her, I placed ethereal crystals on her in the following way:

- Chalcedony on her airways
- Tiger eye on her bronchi
- Tiger Eye and clear quartz in her lungs
- Blue lace agate in her throat
- Chrysocolla in her heart

I knew that she was going to be fine, and the doctor later confirmed this. Her lungs were clear. It would pass.

# Ethereal Crystals and Other Healing Techniques

## Enhancing the Results of Traditional Therapy

### Reiki

Ethereal crystal healing is the next globally known way of healing. Just as reiki came into the mainstream many years ago and is now accepted widely, such will be the case with ethereal crystal healing. What is different from reiki is that with ethereal crystals we also create, but reiki and ethereal crystal healing can easily be combined. By placing ethereal crystals where needed, the reiki healer will receive deeper messages for the client, and the healing will happen faster because the ethereal crystals are changing vibrations in the core.

### Past Life Regression

Ethereal crystals are a beautiful helping hand in any kind of healing. I use them during past life regression and aura and chakra healing as they help release the energy the person is finding it hard to let go of. As people tell me what they're experiencing, I place ethereal crystals on those thoughts in their mind, the energy around them, the connection between that person and the past life experience, in the chakras, and so on. Whatever you feel is needed, place the ethereal crystal there.

## Massage Therapy and Physiotherapy

We are all energy. The body is only a learning tool needed on Earth to be able to do what needs to be done, our life mission. There is too much emphasis on what the body can do. Nothing, is the answer; it is all in the vibration—the body responds to it, and physical life responds to it.

During a massage, ethereal crystals can be placed in tense muscles or places in the body that are "asking for help". They can also be intentionally placed on the chakras so the relaxing massage goes deeper and heals the core issues beneath the painful physical manifestation.

## Aura and Chakra Healing

We wash our physical bodies, so we don't get uncomfortable, smelly, or ill, so why not cleanse our energy system? It catches energies and gathers influences from so many situations and people throughout the day. By placing ethereal crystals, we make sure that vibrations stay high and fresh.

Chakra healing with ethereal crystals can be accomplished in five minutes. The ethereal crystals are placed by intention with the client standing or sitting down. They then get on with their day while the ethereal crystals do their work as long as needed.

## Psychotherapy and Counselling

Psychotherapists can place ethereal crystals in their patients' mind, connections, and situations to help change the vibration and support transformation.

The awareness of humankind is still very much at a turning point, and not everyone is able to release their past and live in full light, love, happiness, and health at this time. This is normal; everything in its own time. Feel deep compassion and love for them, because not long ago you were there, too. At the end of the day, we must start somewhere.

And never forget that whatever ethereal crystals are placed, even when not accepted, they will have a positive effect somewhere, on a different and deeper level; even when the free will declines.

# 23

# Generational Trauma
## Changing the Cycle to Accelerate the Ascension of Humanity and Vibration

Generational trauma—that is, trauma that extends from one genera-tion to the next—begins when a group of individuals experience a traumatic event on economic, religious, cultural, or familial level.

It only takes one survivor to end something that has taken place on such huge scale. We are all vibration; we are all one.

- Awareness
- Changing vibration
- Persistence

Generational trauma carries lessons on a collective consciousness scale. When we break the hold of generational trauma, we heal more than just our family line; we heal the collective vibrations of a generation: shame, hypervigilance, depression, fear, anxiety, sexual abuse, mental abuse, separation, and hate. As long as generational trauma continues, vibrations of separation continue. This is the opposite of who we truly are: love and oneness.

Souls experiencing generational trauma come with the task of expe-riencing oneness. To get there, they must first experience the opposite, as I have done in past lives, and you might have, too, or experienced it in this life. Your soul declared, "I want to experience oneness." But on a human consciousness level, you weren't ready to experience that in a blissful earthly life. It wouldn't have meant anything if you had done. So the Universe gave you the opposite first: separation.

Thus, when someone wakes up and changes the vibration, it positively influences a whole generation on a collective level. We are all helping each other.

A friend of mine was persecuted and had to flee her home country back in the Nineties during a war. Her family settled in a new country, and she fully integrated. After a few years, they were forced to leave their new country, though, and were sent back to their home country. My friend was persecuted, branded a person of no importance, and separated from everyone else, and she and her family and friends experienced separation, anxiety, hypervigilance, PTSD, and war trauma.

But she woke up, healed, and changed her vibration, and thanks to that experience, she now knows what oneness is and helped heal her contemporaries who also experienced the same thing. She is now a successful life coach and multiple gold medallist in her sport, connecting others, one with life and the Universe.

The family of another friend of mine experienced generational sexual trauma during the second world war. Like so many people, her family and their friends had to hide, but the soldiers found them and decided to use the young girls for their pleasure. My friend's grandmother was 12 years old when it happened. Even though my friend had no idea what this generational trauma was until later in life, she struggled her whole life with sexual anxiety and so much more. Then she found out and broke the hold of this generational trauma.

Someone very close to me goes to the refugee camps in Dunkirk, France, every month. There, you will find people from all over the world who have experienced generational trauma. They have fled their countries, travelled soul-destroying journeys to get to Dunkirk, and are waiting there to get on a boat for that last dangerous trip to the UK.

My friend brings food and clothes and offers medical support and a human touch to all who are there. These people do not risk their lives and that of their children for the fun of it. These people make life-threatening journeys out of desperation, to save their lives, to save their children's lives, and to try and find oneness. Even as they undertake these perilous journeys, they experience complete separation as they are persecuted in every way.

Many people feel threatened by refugees. They fear other religions, they fear languages they don't understand, they fear different habits and customs. Refugees trigger old fears in others who react from an old vibrational memory of separation. *There is you, and there is me. I will not accept you breaking through my protective comfort zone.*

People who do not accept refugees live in a similar fear vibration and generational trauma. Some Europeans still carry generational trauma from the first and second world wars, and they fear the separation their grandparents or great-grandparents felt and that refugees are experiencing now. The vibrations from personal experiences in the past are still present and are being triggered by refugees trying to enter their country. In this third-hand generational trauma, it's important we wake up and change the vibration from fear and separation to trust and oneness. If we don't, these vibrations continue and multiply rapidly.

My children are a mix of Belgian and British. We have lived in three different countries while they were growing up: Belgium, Britain, and Ireland.

My daughter said to me one day: "I am too Belgian to be British. I'm too British to be Belgian, and I'm too English to be Irish. Who am I?"

She's experiencing separation so that she can find oneness. Within her separation, she will bring people together.

I answered her by saying: "You are human, a woman of the world. You belong everywhere."

The main message of generational trauma is one of healing separation and hate in order to become what we truly are: oneness and love. If we don't heal this, it continues into the next generation.

All those generational traumas continue to send out their vibrations, mirroring back and forth. We only need one generation without trauma and the healing of generational trauma to return to oneness. Let's all wake up and make changes, whether you're on the active trauma side or the memory vibration side.

We are all one, and our vibrational change will get us there.

# 24

# Creating with Ethereal Crystals

## Creating the Life You Really Want

We are the creators of our physical existence. As soon as we become aware of that, we set in motion a series of actions that cannot be stopped. We can't undo what we learn on our journey as humans; we can only choose to accept or deny the lessons.

The more we choose to accept our lessons, the more other people's trains will be set in motion and the faster all the trains will go. We enter a vortex of conscious creators of life.

Ethereal crystals can be a magical support in creating the life you desire, whether it relates to your health, relationships, money, work, or something else.

Step one is to decide what it is you truly desire and describe it using positive wording, or an affirmation. For example, if you have lung disease, you might say, "I choose and accept the creation of healthy lungs." Or if you want to create a fantastic job, you might say, "I choose and accept the creation of a fun, inspiring job with great colleagues." In other words, focus on the desired result. By doing so, you already shift your vibration. You are choosing and accepting the action that will create the reality.

We have experienced the dark in order to see the light. We're making our journey back to oneness. In the creation process, you are guaranteed to feel jealousy at some point. Until you fully own the fact that everything you desire is yours in divine perfection, jealousy will pop up. Once trust comes in, the vibration of jealousy will no longer be present, because you will know that everything you want to create is yours and better.

Jealousy simply means "I want that, but I haven't got it." Instead, as noted earlier, say, "Yes please!" and choose an ethereal crystal to place in your mind.

This statement will help transform the vibration so that you come in alignment with what you desire, and you can trust that divine timing will bring it to you in the perfect way for you. That may be different from what you expect, but believe me when I say that it will be so perfect for you, you will no longer dwell on what you thought it should look like when the desire first entered your heart.

We are all raised with the belief that we have to work hard to attain happiness. Yet when you love what you do and it is in alignment with your soul purpose, you work hard for the love of it and it doesn't feel "hard".

You cannot find happiness and fulfil your dreams by avoiding pain. The information about ethereal crystals I am sharing in this book has nothing to do with getting rid of pain. Reaching your goals and being happy come from facing and accepting your pain. You have gone through all that pain in order to know what you *don't* want; now you can focus on what you *do* want.

Often during healing and the creation of a new vibration, the old pain pushes forward even more. This is an opportunity for you to heal. Be willing to experience your painful thoughts and feelings without judgement, and to then, with the help of the vibration from a particular ethereal crystal, take inspired action towards your goal. It is that willingness and commitment that will bring the happiness you desire, more happiness than you could have ever imagined possible.

The following list matches ethereal crystals with what they can be used to create:

- **Sodalite:** inner peace, a healthy mind, patience, trust, clairvoyance, a job in travel, the best location to live
- **Smoky quartz:** smoke-free living, clarity, being seen, a career in TV, acting, modelling
- **Clear quartz:** being in the limelight, a practice with lots of clients, a practice as a holistic practitioner, winning prizes
- **Garnet:** money, passion, a healthy heart, ideas

- **Hematite:** power, healthy blood, a powerful sports career, protection
- **Aventurine:** physical beauty, choice, physical attraction, a healthy physical heart, emotional stability
- **Fluorite:** full physical health, miracles, speaking on stage, turnarounds, ascension
- **Topaz:** trauma healing, success, an open door, anything you desire, vacations
- **Turquoise:** safe travel, easy menopause, cancer healing, boundaries, communication, thriving business, friendships
- **Sunstone:** pregnancy, healthy parenting, good weather, healthy eyes and heart, success, sunny relationships, healthy businesses
- **Chrysocolla:** a pain-free life, communication flow, healed relationships, calm after the storm
- **Aquamarine:** parenting through adoption, leadership, successful business, clairvoyance, work/a job, being first, political success bringing positive change
- **Onyx:** healthy hearing, happiness, confidence, healthy relationships
- **Obsidian:** living in the here and now, something new from darkness, transformation
- **Calcite:** healthy bones, success, mental health, a strong physical body, the best possible outcome for you
- **Ruby:** leadership, pregnancy, leadership in sports, business grounding & success, happiness
- **Jasper:** a healthy physical head, pregnancy, creating who you desire to be in full alignment with your soul's purpose, a home, a house
- **Rose quartz:** a healed childhood, a beautiful childhood, self-love, love relationships, healthy breasts, heart, & blood, effective parenting, patience
- **Agate:** perfect health, healthy sexual relationships, enlightenment, fearlessness, rhythm instead of chaos, a healthy childhood, a medical profession, a perfect mentor
- **Chalcedony:** flow, riverside property, travel, emotional control, close bonds
- **Lapis Lazuli:** wonderful friendships, new ideas/solutions, happiness, success as a teacher

- **Amethyst:** freedom from addiction, clarity, a home with good feng shui, clutter-free relationships
- **Emerald:** love relationships, contracts, agreements, spiritual growth & practices
- **Malachite:** femininity, being, pregnancy, a new job, sexuality, sexual enjoyment, gentleness
- **Labradorite:** a property development portfolio, career in architecture, success in anything to do with building & property, a career in counselling & guidance
- **Tourmaline:** fixing electrical appliances, careers in mechanics and electrical engineering, careers in supporting and caring for older & vulnerable people, careers in policing & safeguarding, IT
- **Moonstone:** career as a midwife, career in women's healthcare, including their hormones/sexuality/emotions, career as an emotional guide, mentor, or counsellor, weight loss, generational change
- **Unakite:** wealth, abundance, money, fame, generational healing, release of shackles in any way, healing from war trauma, healing from substance abuse, healing from religious trauma, healing generational trauma
- **Tiger eye:** shamanism/witchcraft practice, protection, a career in fashion, healthy pregnancy
- **Sphalerite:** a new body and mind, rehabilitation after coma, paralysis, loss of movement, brain damage, connection with the body, healthy muscles, a career in bodybuilding and gymnastics
- **Morganite:** a career in motor sports, a career in anything linked to speed and movement, a career in horse racing or as an equestrian, ancestral healing, multiple relationships with investors, collaborations, and sponsors
- **Amber:** a career related to beauty, perfect health
- **Citrine:** work as an extra on a film, a career in a creative industry (film, publishing, journalism), a successful home and family life.

We are all different. However, just as single flowers gathered into a bunch become a beautiful, fragrant bouquet, our individuality can be a united force when we realize we become whole when gathered together.

# Suggested Resources

Most of this book was channelled. I received the information about how to work with ethereal crystals over 10 years ago from my spirit guide. I knew I had to write about ethereal crystals, but the specifics came later. I asked the Universe, "What needs to be written in this book?" and Part One and the rest is what came through.

For those interested in exploring further, I recommend the following:

## Books

Delanote, Marie. *The Healing of the 1lb Baby*. New York: Clink Street Publishing, 2014. My first book documents the birth and healing of my extremely premature daughter.

———. *Acorns to Great Oaks: Meditations for Children*. Book and CD. Scotland: Findhorn Press, 2017. Twenty-two meditations to help children manage their emotions.

———. *Ethereal Crystals Healing Oracle Deck*. 2022. Available from www.mariedelanote.net. Free shipping worldwide. This companion deck draws on the specific messages of ethereal crystals and offers daily guidance to your questions.

Dispenza, Joe. *You Are the Placebo: Making Your Mind Matter*. Carlsbad, CA: Hay House, 2014. Stories of healing that show beautifully how you are the creator of your own life.

Emoto, Masaru. *The Miracle of Water*. New York: Atria, 2007. Late Japanese researcher Dr. Emoto used high-speed microscopic photography to study the effects of positive and negative messages on water crystals. His books underscore the message of my work: It is all about vibration.

Hay, Louise L. *Heal Your Body*. Carlsbad, CA: Hay House, 1981. This ground-breaking classic explores the energetic meaning of physical illnesses.

Honda, Ken. *Happy Money: The Japanese Art of Making Peace with Your Money*. London, UK: John Murray Learning, imprint of Hodder & Stoughton, 2020. A great explanation of the need to balance giving and receiving, and how growing your awareness and raising your vibration can improve your finances.

## CDs

I recommend the following meditation CDs by Dr. Joe Dispenza, which are all available through his website: www.drjoedispenza.com. They are a powerful tool in helping you transcend physical boundaries:

*Changing Boxes: A Guided Meditation*. Rainier, WA: Encephalon, 2019.
*Conditioning Your Body to a New Mind: Walking Meditation*. Rainier, WA: Encephalon, 2018.
*Space Time, Time Space: A Guided Meditation*. Rainier, WA: Encephalon, 2017.
*The Pineal Gland: Tuning into Higher Dimensions of Time and Space: A Guided Meditation*. Rainier, WA: Encephalon, 2017.

## Online

The information about physical crystals in this book came from a course I took with Valerie Truyts in Belgium. I further developed my crystal knowledge—how they work and how they are connected to everything I describe in the book—through working with them myself and with my clients.

*Valerie's Aroma Atelier*. Gemstones, aromatherapy, aura-soma, aura sprays, and online courses and workshops by Valerie Truyts. Courses are in Dutch. www.aroma-atelier.be

# Acknowledgements

Nothing is done by just one individual, and in my case, a long line of masters, teachers, and inspiring individuals have brought me to the place I am now.

Thanks go out to my spiritual guide, who introduced me to ethereal crystals. I am forever grateful for all of the wise masters who came onto my path, pushing me forward towards the next consciousness, so I could gather wisdom, knowledge, and self-love and share them with others.

A special mention to my angels and guides and higher self for being infinitely patient with me, human Marie, while she at times procrastinated and wallowed in self-pity and fear.

I extend deep gratitude to my community of transformational leaders at ATL Europe and our founder Marie Diamond. When I joined, I came home. I am grateful for the support, guidance, and love—so much love.

I would like to thank all the souls that have crossed my path and given me the opportunity to learn and grow. I would also like to thank those who crossed my path in less pleasant situations. Without you, I wouldn't have found my own light and strength.

I would like to acknowledge Els Devogelaere, for the beautiful photographs she created, and Jane Solomon from Biofield Imaging.

I would like to thank my husband who has given me the freedom, opportunity, and space to heal, develop, learn, and grow. I'd like to believe this wasn't just a gift to me but a gift to the whole world.

Finally, I want to express my deepest gratitude to my children. Without them, I wouldn't be where I am now. My biggest teachers of love, and self-love and the guinea pigs for my ethereal crystal healing!

*Thank you,* Marie

# About the Photographer

## Els Devogelaere
*Energy Mentor and Spiritual Photographer*

For more than 30 years, Els has passed on her knowledge and passion for creation, transformation, photography, arts and crafts, and sculpture to thousands of youngsters during her career as an art teacher and photographer.

Her parents taught her the power of positive thinking, and from a young age, she has walked the spiritual path, which has now enabled her to pass on her services as an energy mentor to others.

For more than 25 years, she studied with Marie Diamond, feng shui master and master teacher of The Secret (www.mariediamond.com), who says about Els' work:

With her photographs of crystals, Els Devogelaere brings their transformational energy into expression. Her passion, knowledge, and contact with the energy of the crystals help her pass on the spiritual vibrations to the reader. A truly unique spiritual photographer.

Els' love of crystals prompted her to look at those magnificent light beings on a deeper level, and by looking through the eye of her camera, create a new dimension as a contribution to the evolution of Earth.

Els lives in Belgium, West Flanders, and is mother to Laura and Indy. For more about her work, visit **www.artofearth-chi.be**.

# About the Author

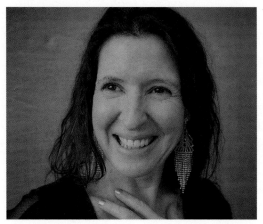

Photo by Carrowmore Photography

Ethereal crystals master and award-winning writer and producer **Marie Delanote** was born in Flanders, Belgium, and moved to Ireland in 2020. Before committing to a career as a writer and filmmaker, Marie pursued a musical vocation, playing the double bass at the Royal Opera House in Belgium. She stopped playing professionally when she decided to be a full-time mum to her four children.

Marie's first book, *The Healing of the 1lb Baby,* about the extremely premature birth of her daughter, was published in 2014 and attracted widespread media attention in the UK and US. Her second book and accompanying CD, *Acorns to Great Oaks: Meditations for Children,* was published in 2017 by Findhorn Press.

Along with producing transformational films, Marie continues to write mind-body-spirit books. As an ethereal crystals master, she offers private sessions and online courses to help people connect with the intelligence and guidance of ethereal crystals to transform energy between people, the physical body, mind, buildings, earth, past lives, and family circles.

Marie is the founder of Ethereal Crystals Global, a company that sells products empowered with ethereal crystals designed to transform energy—physically, emotionally, spiritually, and mentally. She is a proud member of ATL Europe (the Association of Transformational Leaders).

For more about Marie's work visit **www.mariedelanote.net**.

FINDHORN PRESS

Life-Changing Books

Learn more about us and our books at
**www.findhornpress.com**

For information on the Findhorn Foundation:
**www.findhorn.org**

Scan the QR code and save 25% at InnerTraditions.com.
Browse over 2,000 titles on spirituality, the occult, ancient
mysteries, new science, holistic health, and natural medicine.